Praise for

# THE BRAIN FOG FIX

"A vital and scientific manual for the lifestyle choices that can prevent and reverse brain fog."

— **Daniel Amen, M.D.**, *New York Times* best-selling author of *Change Your Brain, Change Your Life*

"Say good-bye to the toxic junk that gunks up your glorious brain. Thank you for this super simple program, Mike! It will leave folks feeling happier, healthier, and more luminous than ever."

— **Kris Carr,** *New York Times* best-selling author of *Crazy Sexy Kitchen*

"An eye-opening look at the way your diet can either promote or prevent brain fog."

— **J. J. Virgin,** *New York Times* best-selling author of *JJ Virgin's Sugar Impact Diet* and *The Virgin Diet*

"If you want to improve your energy and mood, Dr. Mike's program will show you the way."

— **Jackie Warner,** *New York Times* best-selling author of *This Is Why You're Sick and Tired*

"Sugar and inactivity don't just lead to belly fat; they damage the brain. Dr. Mike's plan helps readers revitalize their lives."

— **Jorge Cruise,** *New York Times* best-selling author of *The Belly Fat Cure*™

"Constant blood sugar spikes lead to diabetes . . . and also depression, dementia, and Alzheimer's disease. *The Brain Fog Fix* gives you simple ways to prevent disease and protect your brain."

— **Jorge Rodriguez, M.D.,** author of *The Diabetes Solution*

"Dr. Mike makes understanding our brain chemistry simple yet empowering. This book is a must read for anyone wanting freedom from 'bad brain' plus an escape from the emotional roller coaster our brain chemistry creates. Follow his 21-day plan and rediscover greater energy and joy for life!"

— **Andrea Pennington, M.D.,** author of *The Pennington Plan*

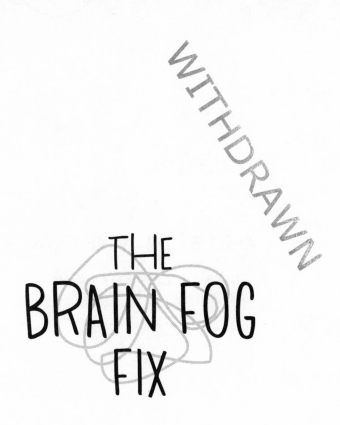

# THE
# BRAIN FOG
# FIX

# ALSO BY DR. MIKE DOW

*Diet Rehab: 28 Days to Finally Stop
Craving the Foods That Make You Fat*

# THE
# BRAIN FOG
# FIX

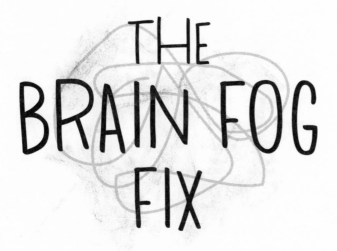

## Reclaim Your Focus, Memory, and Joy in Just 3 Weeks

# DR. MIKE DOW

**HAY HOUSE, INC.**
Carlsbad, California • New York City
London • Sydney • Johannesburg
Vancouver • Hong Kong • New Delhi

*Published and distributed in the United States by:* Hay House, Inc.: www.hayhouse.com® • *Published and distributed in Australia by:* Hay House Australia Pty. Ltd.: www.hayhouse.com.au • *Published and distributed in the United Kingdom by:* Hay House UK, Ltd.: www.hayhouse.co.uk • *Published and distributed in the Republic of South Africa by:* Hay House SA (Pty), Ltd.: www.hayhouse.co.za • *Distributed in Canada by:* Raincoast Books: www.raincoast.com • *Published in India by:* Hay House Publishers India: www.hayhouse.co.in

*Cover & interior design:* Tricia Breidenthal

**Library of Congress Cataloging-in-Publication Data**

Dow, Mike.
   The brain fog fix : reclaim your focus, memory, and joy in just 3 weeks / Dr. Mike Dow. -- 1st edition.
      pages cm
   ISBN 978-1-4019-4647-0 (hardback)
1. Brain--Popular works. 2. Mental health--Popular works. 3. Nutrition--Popular works. 4. Self-care, Health--Popular works. I. Title.
   QP376.D693 2015
   612.8--dc23
                                2015004735

Hardcover ISBN: 978-1-4019-4647-0

10  9  8  7  6  5  4  3
1st edition, September 2015

Printed in the United States of America

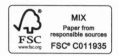

Dad, I hope this book
helps carry the torch you lit
with your life's work in
helping people heal.

Brett, I wish your earthly life
had included more days;
I'm also happy you fully lived
the ones you had here.

# CONTENTS

# INTRODUCTION

*The Brain Fog Fix* is a book about taking better care of your brain to help fight anxiety, depression, brain fog, scatterbrain, and other conditions that are becoming the scary status quo in our country. But it's also a book about using simple strategies to help make your life easier, happier, and more fulfilling. It's all connected: if your brain is in bad shape, chances are the rest of your life is, too.

I wrote this for people like my friend Jane, who considers herself generally happy but doesn't understand why she's always so moody. I wrote it for a patient I recently treated who felt stressed out all the time but didn't have the time to go on a meditation retreat or the financial freedom to quit her job.

I also wrote this book for my grandpa, who followed my advice to eat more berries and keep on traveling to ward off senior moments, and my mom, who regained her lost energy only *after* she weaned herself off the ten (yes, ten!) Diet Cokes she'd gotten into the habit of drinking every single day. I wrote it for my little brother, who co-founded an organization called Aphasia Recovery Connection and, through helping other stroke survivors, has discovered how a sense of purpose can reshape every aspect of life.

I also wrote this book for me.

Even after ten years of practicing cognitive behavioral therapy, I still sometimes fall prey to down periods when I fail to utilize the very strategies I teach. In fact, I conducted an unintentional case study on myself a few years ago, an experiment in how *not* to get through the rocky patches of life. At the time, I was going through a painful break-up while trying to juggle my private practice, finish my first book, and work on some new TV projects. I felt completely overwhelmed, and I found it difficult to think clearly. And most of all I felt incredibly sad.

The problem was not the sadness itself. It was that I allowed the sadness to change my behavior and, in the process, rule (and ruin) my whole life. My primarily pescetarian diet—which consisted of wild salmon, healthy grains, and organic vegetables—gave way to pizza, turkey sandwiches, and ice cream. More often than I'd care to admit, I stayed up watching TV till 3 A.M., then slept till noon. Other evenings I'd stay out way too late drinking, then need five or six big cups of coffee to get through the following day. After feeling exhausted all day, I'd have trouble falling asleep at night.

My workout regimen went from saintly to almost nonexistent. I abandoned the spiritual practices like prayer, meditation, and yoga that have kept me grounded for decades. And instead of connecting with friends and family, I rarely made plans. I still somehow managed to fulfill all my work obligations, but inside I felt confused, unmoored, and generally depressed. The excess drinking, coffee, overeating, isolation, and even a brief stint on Xanax were all just Band-Aids that made my predicament worse, not better.

What should have been a few rough weeks turned into a few *months* of low-grade misery. I learned the hard way that the times in our lives when we *most* need to take care of ourselves often tend to be the times when we're *least* likely to do so. It's easy to show up at yoga class when you feel great, but it's far more important to show up when you feel horrible.

When I finally emerged from that difficult transition, I resolved never to let myself go like that again. I vowed to always practice what I preach, no matter what obstacles life placed in my path.

That decision has helped me immeasurably, on many levels. Since then, I've weathered some other storms, as we all do. Last year I lost my dad and a very dear friend within a few months of each other. Continuing to take good care of myself didn't eradicate the pain: I cried daily when I was grieving, but this time I didn't let the sadness make me abandon the way I want to live.

I've learned that storms pass. You can either be the person who stays inside and boards up the windows during the worst of the rain, or you can be the person who doesn't even bother to swim when waves threaten to wash you out to sea. I hope this book helps teach you to be the former.

The good news is that strengthening your inner reserves is probably easier than you think. Instead of trying to ambitiously overhaul *one* aspect of your life entirely with some difficult-to-maintain resolution, begin by making *small and achievable* changes in many different areas of your life. I take this approach in this book because if I've learned one thing from the thousands of people I've treated, it's that you have to take the whole person into account if you want to think and feel better.

This includes the way you sleep. The way you eat. The way you connect. The way you disconnect. The way you move. The way you love. The way you find peace. The way you remember who you really are.

As you work your way through this book, you'll see that easy changes can create a profound difference in your life. You'll learn that walnuts and grass-fed meats can improve your mood and that one inexpensive spice can drastically reduce your chance of dementia. You'll learn that relationships are more potent than any prescription mood booster and that our use of social media has the power to either improve or erode those relationships. You'll discover how meditation and prayer work in the brain and why spiritual practice isn't an optional extracurricular activity but, rather, a fundamental part of being human. At the end, you'll find a simple 21-day program that will help you put these theories—and many others—into practice as part of your daily life.

When you get out of bed tomorrow morning, you'll make millions of seemingly insignificant choices from the second you wake up. These tiny choices send ripples through time and space. They will affect your body, the way you think, the way you feel, the way you behave, the relationships you're in, and the difference you make in this world.

My hope in writing this book is to teach you how to make all of these seemingly insignificant choices meaningful, which will then help you think and feel a little better tomorrow.

In good health,
Dr. Mike Dow

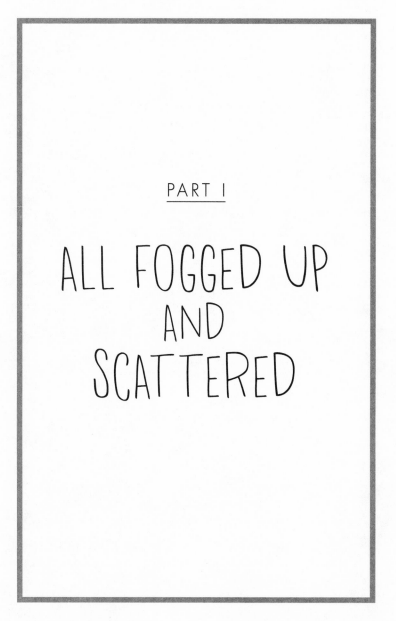

PART I

# ALL FOGGED UP AND SCATTERED

# "I Just Don't Feel Like Myself"

Marin was a 35-year-old physical therapist whose mother had recently been diagnosed with early-onset Alzheimer's. In the tumultuous months that followed, Marin had been facing all the challenges of getting her beloved mother's affairs in order while struggling with the anguish of watching her drift deeper and deeper into dementia.

Marin thought that she was handling her situation as well as possible, but she also felt that she was "in a slump."

"I wake up exhausted every morning," she told me, "yet I can't sleep at night. Most of the time, I'm just dragging myself through the day."

When I asked Marin what in her life gave her pleasure, she just shrugged.

"I used to enjoy my job," she said, "but now I'm just going through the motions. I had a boyfriend, but after all this stuff started with my mother, I got depressed and we broke up. I don't blame Tony," she told me, shrugging again. "I wouldn't have wanted to go out with me, either."

When I asked Marin how she spent her time away from work, she had to think for a moment. "It feels like I'm always at work," she finally told me. "Especially now that Tony's out of the picture, there's just not the same incentive to get out of the office at a reasonable hour. I don't know . . . I guess when I get home I go on Facebook. Or watch a little TV. Twitter, of course, and Instagram. And I thought maybe if I went on Tinder, I'd find a new guy, but I haven't really liked anyone. So probably mainly Facebook. It's a great way to keep up with people, isn't it? But it does take up a lot of time."

As we continued to talk, Marin seemed to become more and more tired. "It's always like this," she said bleakly. "I just don't have any energy unless there's a crisis. When I get a call about Mom, somehow I find a way to muscle through the problem. But for anything else . . . I don't know. I just feel like I'm in a permanent fog."

☐

Karen was a retired teacher in her late 50s who had been divorced for three years. She came to see me a few months after her second child had graduated from high school and left for college.

"I thought I was finally going to have time for myself," she told me. "With the kids out of the house and Philip gone, I expected a whole new life to begin. I thought I'd start dating again, get back to painting, maybe take a salsa class or start ballroom dancing. I had so many wonderful plans. But now I just sit at home every night watching television, and I think, *What's the point?*"

When Karen consulted her doctor about her "dragginess," as she put it, he prescribed an antidepressant. Karen thought the medication was helping her feel fewer lows, but she also felt like she felt fewer highs. She still had no motivation to go out and meet new people or explore any of the activities she had fantasized about during her years of raising kids. She felt lonely and bored and seldom even left the house. What was happening to her?

## UNDERSTANDING BRAIN FOG

A new epidemic is sweeping the country—an epidemic of many names.

Some people call it brain fog.

Some people call it depression.

Some call it ADHD (attention-deficit hyperactivity disorder), scatterbrain, or an inability to focus.

And some people simply say they just don't feel like themselves—and haven't for a long time.

We mental health professionals may refer to these vague conditions as "chronic cognitive and mood problems." But the clinical jargon doesn't begin to evoke the frustration, anxiety, and downright misery experienced by the millions of people whose brains are simply not working properly.

My primary job as a cognitive behavioral therapist is to help my patients transform their thoughts and feelings, and the best way to do this is to help them change their behavior. Whether they're learning to ride a bike or falling in love for the first time, human beings are most dramatically changed by their own experiences.

I wanted to help Marin and Karen—and many others who came to me with similar complaints—figure out how to tackle the unique challenges they were facing. I wanted to help them develop the coping skills and perspective to make satisfying decisions, endure what they could not change, and savor as much of life as possible. I knew that the insights I had gained through my professional experience could help them think more clearly and feel better, and I was eager to share all my resources.

But I also knew that their problems were not just emotional. Biology was at play, too. Many of my patients had significant imbalances in their brain chemistry—imbalances that were seriously interfering with their ability to experience their power, joy, and purpose. Spirituality, connection, and social elements needed to be addressed, too, since treating the whole person is key to lasting change.

For most, these imbalances didn't require prescription medication—only a handful of them would have been diagnosed with depression. Nor were most of these problems chronic; all of these patients could recall long periods of time when they had been able to think clearly and felt great. Unfortunately, many of their diets, lifestyles, and circumstances were conspiring to destabilize their brain chemistry, leaving them thinking badly and feeling worse.

My patients were suffering because of their imbalanced, under-nourished brains—and they were by no means alone. Far too many of us are in the same situation. Just consider these alarming statistics for a sobering sense of the state of brain health in this country:

- According to the U.S. Department of Health and Human Services, only 17 percent of American adults are considered to be in a state of "optimal mental health."[1]

- One American adult in ten takes some kind of medication to cope with depression. In American women in their 40s and 50s, that number is one in four. And one in five Americans takes a prescription drug for a psychiatric illness.

- Along with depression, anxiety is also on the rise. Xanax is the country's most prescribed psychiatric drug, even though studies have shown that it may shrink the brain in the same way long-term alcohol abuse does.

- Some 10 to 15 percent of U.S. adults suffer from insomnia, and according to the CDC, 50 million Americans report an insufficient amount of sleep. Sales of both over-the-counter and prescription sleep aids are skyrocketing.

- Overdose deaths from prescription painkillers have tripled over the past ten years.

- Thirty-eight million U.S. adults drink too much (CDC).

- ADHD diagnosis rates are through the roof. They've already tripled in children, and stimulant abuse is rising rapidly as more and more high school and college students are scoring Adderall to party or enhance performance.

- Prescription rates of antipsychotic medications have doubled in the U.S. over the past ten years.

- More than 5 million people in the United States are living with Alzheimer's, and according to the Alzheimer's Association, up to 16 million Americans will suffer from the disease by 2050.

- More than 35 million people worldwide are currently living with dementia. By 2050, that number is expected to more than triple to a staggering 115 million.

- Many millions more are suffering from the condition known as mild neurocognitive disorder, which is similar to subjective cognitive impairment or mild cognitive impairment—all diagnoses for brains that aren't working properly but don't qualify for a diagnosis of dementia.

Depression. Anxiety. Sleeplessness. Forgetfulness. Confusion. Dementia.

In so many ways, many of us are thinking and feeling worse than ever. Why?

The short answer is that our brains are simply not getting the support they need to produce the essential brain chemicals that keep us energized, calm, focused, and inspired. In fact, if you look at the way most of us live, it's almost as though we have chosen a lifestyle deliberately intended to undermine our brain chemistry.

If you gorge yourself constantly on donuts, ice cream, bacon, and fried chicken, you will almost certainly gain weight. In the same way, if you eat the wrong foods, get insufficient exercise or sleep, overindulge in social media and TV, have too much stress and too little downtime, and cope with loneliness and lack of connection and meaning, you will almost certainly disrupt your brain chemistry. It really is that simple—and that painful.

The inevitable result of this chronically imbalanced brain chemistry is cognitive and mood problems (i.e., thinking badly and feeling worse). And at the moment, just about everything in our current lives serves to unbalance and undermine our brains. Our brains don't get what they require to maintain high levels of the feel-good brain chemicals *serotonin* and *dopamine* and low levels of the stress hormone *cortisol*.

Instead, we haze, daze, and wire our brains with caffeine, sugar, starches, electronics, distractions, and unnecessary stress—a recipe virtually guaranteed to disrupt our brain chemistry. And then we rely on short-term Band-Aids like excessive caffeine, antidepressants, sleep aids, and social isolation that ultimately exacerbate our problems.

The good news is that you can reverse these trends and take charge of your brain health without too much difficulty at all. I'll show you how.


## THE BRAIN DRAIN

As a scientist and mental health professional who has studied the complexities of the human brain for years, I can come to only one conclusion. The way we eat, sleep, work, and live is flooding, starving, clogging, and disrupting our brains by destabilizing the levels of three crucial brain chemicals: *serotonin, dopamine,* and *cortisol.* We experience these biological problems as brain fog, scatterbrain, memory loss, fatigue, anxiety, and the blues. Over time, they turn into chronic insomnia, significant depression, persistent anxiety, and, potentially, dementia.

To make matters worse, the conventional response to these problems is actually creating even bigger problems. Insomnia makes us tired, so we turn to caffeine and energy drinks, which keep us from sleeping, which in turn lead us to seek over-the-counter or prescription sleep aids. The sleeping pills produce residual drowsiness, so we awaken feeling listless and unfocused and inevitably drink even *more* caffeine.

Over time, our mood worsens and our brain fogs, so we seek out antidepressants and perhaps some Adderall and yet more caffeine to help improve our focus. Then we need antianxiety meds and that extra glass of wine to calm ourselves down after all the stimulants we've ingested. All of these medications create side effects of their own, including weight gain, lowered sex drive, and, in some cases, chemical dependence.

Unfortunately, far too many people view these problems as distinct and unrelated. We see a dietician to lose weight; we consult a psychiatrist for mood problems; we take a sleeping pill for insomnia. But recent groundbreaking research has shown that physical, psychological, social, and spiritual health are even more intricately connected than we previously imagined.

Take our diet: we now know that keeping blood sugar low isn't just good for weight loss; it also makes the brain work faster and prevents brain fog. Meditation or prayer isn't just for monks or for people who want to find God; it also improves memory, mood, and attention span. Depression isn't just about low serotonin or dopamine that can be corrected only with prescription medication; it's also about our brains needing more anti-inflammatory foods and experiences that promote neurogenesis, or the growth of new brain cells and connections. What's good for the body is also good for the brain—and the soul, too.

Unfortunately, far too many of us are eating blood sugar–spiking carbohydrates and high omega-6 proteins and fats at every snack and meal, both of which can affect mood and intelligence and even set us up for dementia, which generally first surfaces as brain fog or scatterbrain—problems that we might've avoided simply by taking better care of our brains and bodies.

Even if you *think* you're eating a super-healthy diet of grilled chicken breast, egg whites, "fresh" (but farm-raised) salmon, and nonfat Greek yogurt, your brain is being undermined by the invisible changes in your food supply. Just a few generations ago, almost all farms were family owned and operated. They're now predominantly gigantic factory farms that pump their cows and chickens full of cheap feed that doesn't just change the animals' health—it changes yours as well.

Environmental pollutants like mercury and BPAs can also affect the health of our brains, and fundamental changes in our lifestyle and environment play a vital role as well. For the first time in American history, people are more likely to live alone than with a significant other. There are fewer lasting marriages and more divorces than in previous times.

Despite greater connectivity through social media, we are actually becoming more isolated. Single people spending more and more time alone in their apartments in front of their computers and televisions makes the problem worse. Facebook friend numbers are up, but closeness in actual flesh-and-blood friendships is down.

Some of this constant connectivity has started to feel mandatory. Since we're no longer working for one company for 30 years with a great pension plan to help us through our retirement, we'd better make sure our LinkedIn profile is up-to-date just in case another downsizing is on the horizon. With all these stresses in our lives, many of us have neglected to pursue any spiritual and/or religious practice. We spend so much time "doing" that we have forgotten how important simply "being," or "nondoing," is for the brain.

Before beginning work on this book, I knew that we were facing widespread problems. But when I looked at the numbers, I came to see that these challenges to the brain actually constitute a full-blown epidemic—one that the conventional health-care system is inadvertently making worse. Instead of steering us toward simple diet and lifestyle changes, healing spiritual practices, and human connections that actually support our brain health, we're taught to rely on drugs, which tend to disrupt our brain chemistry even further.

If there is another way to care for our brains—a natural approach drawing on nutrition, exercise, sleep, meditation, and lifestyle—shouldn't we choose that over medications that produce troubling side effects and possibly dangerous long-term consequences? Shouldn't we at least try? Of course, some people desperately need pharmaceutical help, usually in the short run, sometimes over the long term. But a shockingly large number of people are being given meds they really do not need to address problems that would be better solved in other ways.

For example, nearly one out of ten Americans takes antidepressants, yet a recent large-scale study showed that nearly two-thirds of these people did not fit the clinical definition of "depressed," making these medications a questionable choice at best. Yes, these people likely felt foggy, listless, unmotivated, or blue. And yes, they likely had real problems that required real help. But before trying Prozac, did they try anything else? Anything more natural?

In this book I'll teach you how to address the big picture: your diet, your sleeping schedule, and the everyday lifestyle choices that may be more dangerous than you realize. Every time we skip the gym and stay up late watching TV, answering e-mail, and working on the computer; every time we turn to social media instead of connecting face-to-face with our loved ones, we set ourselves up for depression, anxiety, scatterbrain, and brain fog. Our sedentary lives are softening our bodies and depriving our brains of the hormones they need to thrive, and our 24/7 technology addiction is starving us of sleep and alienating us from the people we love.

If you want to lead a fulfilling and inspiring life, you have to begin by restoring your normal levels of *serotonin, dopamine,* and *cortisol,* the three hormones that are most essential to thinking and feeling your best. Making some remarkably simple changes will allow you to rebalance your brain chemistry and tap into your inner reserves of power, joy, and purpose.

# CHAPTER 2

# It's Not You— It's Your Brain!

Let's delve a little deeper into why you have been feeling so gloomy and draggy, or just forgetful and uninspired—and, more important, what you can do to fix it.

Think about what a typical day is like for many of us.

The alarm goes off, jarring you out of a restless sleep. You wake up tired and lackluster, but before you've even gotten out of bed, you reach for your phone, and before you know it, your heart is racing at the influx of texts, Tweets, and e-mails that have accumulated overnight. Maybe you answer a few e-mails, or maybe you just make some mental notes with a slowly growing sense of Monday-morning dread, but either way, you're already in work mode, your mind dashing from one demand to the next.

You don't feel rested or energized, let alone focused, so you reach for some caffeine to help get you out of the house. If you have kids, you're rushing around trying to make sure they eat their breakfast and have lunches, permission slips, textbooks, gym clothes—what else have you forgotten? You skip breakfast altogether, or perhaps you grab a breakfast pastry or a piece of toast. Maybe you even choose a deceptively marketed "heart-healthy, whole-grain" cereal bar.

You race off to work, your mind buzzing with a million obliga-tions—talk to your boss about that conference, don't forget to buy milk on the way home, call your mom about Sunday dinner, make a doctor's appointment for your daughter . . .

Once you get to your desk, you hit the ground running, checking your e-mail while simultaneously returning calls and texts, plunging into the tasks that have piled up overnight. Just a generation ago, business was rarely conducted after 6 P.M., but now, with the 24-hour electronic cycle, tasks accumulate around the clock so you almost never feel caught up, even when you come in early.

Throughout the day, you rarely have more than a few minutes to work without interruption. Calls, e-mails, texts, instant messages, and other electronic demands are constantly coming in, and even when they don't actively interrupt you, you have learned to interrupt yourself—breaking off a conversation to return a text, pausing in the midst of a task to compulsively check your e-mail. Most of your con-versations are electronic—and short. You can't get into much detail in 140 characters.

You might also jump onto Facebook several times a day, trying to keep up with the lives of your many friends, though you can't help resenting how thin and glowing Sonya always looks—why can't *you* lose weight? Your friend Jane is always posting about her latest ro-mantic prospect—why don't *you* ever have that kind of fun? Marisela's kids always seem so happy and composed—why are *your* kids so hard to handle?

Lunch is likely rushed, and caffeine is likely frequent. If you do have time for a snack during the day, you might grab a cookie or maybe even a virtuous granola bar, not realizing that both the "healthy" and the "unhealthy" snacks are packed with carbs and sugars, and not enough of the amino acids, vitamins, and omega-3s that your brain needs to function optimally.

You might have to stay late at work, but even if you leave on time, you often take work home with you. You'll check your e-mail at least every half hour, answer a business call, or return a text—maybe even a constant flow of texts.

When was the last time you had a truly relaxing, restorative dinner that left you feeling nourished, satisfied, and deeply connected to the people you love? Maybe you've squeezed in a half hour for the gym or the exercise bike, but it's a rare day when you have time to sit quietly, savor the moment, see something beautiful, or feel yourself flooded with peace and contentment. Electronic evenings are crammed with simultaneous Twitter, texting, Facebook, e-mail, and TV, none of which are likely to absorb your full attention or leave you feeling fulfilled.

When it comes time to fall asleep, perhaps you find yourself wired and wakeful, your mind still racing with the items that you haven't yet ticked off your never-ending to-do list, the tasks you haven't finished. Maybe you take a sleeping pill, knowing that it won't give you the restful sleep you crave but grateful for at least the chance to turn off for the day. And then tomorrow the whole crazy cycle starts right up again . . .

## GETTING YOUR BRAIN BACK IN BALANCE

Don't panic! There *is* a solution, and implementing it is far easier than you might think.

Our brains rely on a complex symphony of chemicals to keep our moods in check and to function properly. Our brains are equipped to learn a new language, rise to a challenge, enjoy an exciting adventure, or just relax contentedly in a hammock.

But when our brain chemicals get out of whack, all sorts of problems can arise. We can become depressed, or be unable to sleep, or be too riled up to concentrate. We can feel over-the-top ecstatic one minute and completely despondent the next. We can forget where we put our wallet or feel too exhausted to walk out the door—all because our brains are getting the wrong quantities of chemicals.

As I noted in the last chapter, the three brain chemicals most responsible for thinking and feeling are *serotonin, dopamine,* and *cortisol,* and the ultimate goal of this program is to get them back in balance.

*Serotonin* is primarily responsible for feelings of calm, serenity, optimism, and self-confidence. When you feel as though all's right with the world, it's your serotonin levels that are at work. When you feel hopeful about a project being successful, a job interview going well, or a big effort paying off, your serotonin levels are probably healthy. If your serotonin levels are low, you might experience depression, anxiety, hopelessness, sleep problems, a negative attitude, and lack of self-confidence.

*Not enough serotonin → vulnerability to physical and emotional pain → painkillers, antidepressants, and antianxiety meds → brain fog, reduced sexual function, possible dependence*

*Dopamine* is the chemical basis for feeling excited, motivated, energized, and "pleasured." Dopamine allows you to enjoy the intense fun and excitement of riding a roller coaster, winning a big race, falling in love, or even going on a shopping spree. When life seems engaging, interesting, and enjoyable, your dopamine levels are likely in good shape. Low dopamine levels can result in listlessness, boredom, and the general sense that life has lost its savor. Imbalanced dopamine can also make it harder to focus, to think things through, and to control your impulses. Imbalanced dopamine is associated with compulsive and addictive behavior of all types—from cocaine addition to compulsive shopping—as well as ADHD.

*Imbalanced dopamine → feeling unfocused, unmotivated, bored, impulsive → risky activities, caffeine, stimulants, Adderall → "crashes" from the highs, brain fog, listlessness, possible dependence*

*Cortisol* is the stress hormone that your body uses to rev into high gear. You need a little cortisol to meet all the large and small demands that life throws at you. Imbalanced cortisol levels can leave you feeling exhausted, wired, or sometimes both: listless and dragged out during the day, anxious and sleepless at night. When your cortisol levels are off balance, you might feel so frayed that the smallest problem sets you off, or so unmotivated that you can barely drag yourself through the day—or, in many cases, both. Permanently high cortisol can depress dopamine levels while preventing serotonin from binding to certain areas in your brain. High cortisol levels have also been shown to inhibit neurogenesis—the creation of new brain cells.

*Imbalanced cortisol → feeling exhausted, wired, or both → caffeine, sleep aids, sometimes antidepressants or antianxiety meds → brain fog, increased problems of exhaustion and sleeplessness, sexual side effects, anxiety, depression → possible dependence*

Here's the bottom line: no matter what you're going through—minor stress, an uninspiring life, a major crisis, or a course of chemotherapy—the key to feeling better lies in rebalancing these three brain chemicals.

And that's exactly what we're going to do during the 21 days of my program, through a combination of physical, mental, and spiritual approaches.

## BRAIN CHEMISTRY IS THE KEY

Starting with your brain chemistry is crucial, because when your serotonin, dopamine, and cortisol levels are not properly balanced, your brain simply does not work the way it's supposed to. If your brain chemistry is amiss, all the "brain training," psychotherapy, and positive thinking in the world won't cure what ails you.

This is a hard concept for many people to grasp. We often assume that thinking well is a matter of training and willpower, and that feeling great is the result of attitude or life circumstances. But that is a far too simplistic viewpoint.

Obviously, many factors contribute to how well we think and how great we feel. But if our brain chemistry is out of balance, we are unable to think and feel our best. It's just not how we humans are engineered. Thinking and feeling are real experiences you can feel, and they are connected to specific chemical reactions you can see in the brain. If you throw off that chemistry, your brain simply cannot do its job.

Attempting to think and feel great without the proper balance of brain chemicals is like trying to run a marathon with a broken leg. If you were in that condition, working out at the gym wouldn't help. Willpower wouldn't help. New running techniques or those crazy finger-shoes wouldn't help, and neither would an Olympic-caliber coach or the most devoted running buddy in the world. All those things would help only *if* your leg were strong enough to walk on.

So think of these three weeks of brain-chemical balancing as the healing you need to fix that broken leg—only in this case, it's a malnourished and overworked brain. Our healing methods will encompass physical, mental, emotional, and spiritual approaches— because each of these approaches has a significant impact on your brain chemistry.

We will work to give your brain what it needs and remove any obstacles in its way. Because the remarkable thing about your brain is that it is designed to balance its own chemistry—*if* it gets the right nutrients and other support to do so. But when your brain does *not* get what it needs, the rest of your life starts to go haywire. The same thing happens when factors in your life *block* your brain from making the chemicals it needs.

Those are the two core principles underlying this program:

1. Give your brain what it needs.

2. Remove the obstacles that block your brain from optimal function.

Here's a basic breakdown of what exactly your brain needs to thrive—and what is preventing it from doing so.

## What Your Brain Needs

- Proper nutrients, including the right vitamins, essential amino acids, and healthy fats
- Exercise
- Sufficient restful sleep
- Regular, healthy circadian rhythms
- Downtime for relaxation and restoration
- Purpose and meaning
- Spiritual practice
- A connection to something larger than yourself

## What Fogs Your Brain

- Sugar, high-fructose corn syrup, and artificial sweeteners
- Processed white flour
- Too many inflammatory foods, including conventionally grown meat, unhealthy fats, and many artificial ingredients and preservatives
- An imbalance of omega-6 and omega-3 fats
- An excessive use of such brain-altering substances as caffeine, alcohol, and recreational drugs
- Many medications, including unnecessary antidepressants, antianxiety agents, ADHD stimulants, sleep aids, and painkillers
- Overexposure to the "blue light" of electronic screens, including computer, TV, and phone
- Bombardment with diverse tasks and inputs, such as an ongoing flood of social media, texting, Tweeting, Facebooking, Instagramming, and e-mail
- Too much time spent in activities that do not feel meaningful and purposeful, whether they're obligations (such as work and family duties) or entertainment (such as shopping or gambling)

By depriving your brain of the nutrients it needs to balance its own chemistry, you are causing yourself to think badly and feel worse.

By providing your brain with the nutrients it needs, you immediately put yourself on the path to thinking and feeling better.

## A BROKEN-DOWN ENGINE

Let's put our brain health into terms that are easy for everyone to understand. Imagine for a moment that you have a car that is sputtering along at half speed, or has maybe even ground to a halt. You remember the days when this car zipped around smoothly and efficiently, the days when you actively looked forward to taking it out for a spin.

Now, however, your motor is sluggish, your gears creak whenever you speed up, and every mile is an enormous effort. Why?

Maybe you've simply run out of gas. That's an easy fix—add more gas and problem solved!

But perhaps the problem is in your transmission, which lacks the fluid it needs to change gears smoothly. Then the solution would be to add some transmission fluid.

What if there is a little hole in the brake lining, so that all the brake fluid is draining away? Then you have two problems: you need to add more brake fluid *and* you need to fix the hole that is causing the leak.

Suppose your battery is dead, or dying . . . or your tires are rapidly losing air . . . or the computer that governs your car has stopped working properly.

Any or all of these issues might be keeping your car from running optimally. And until you have brought them *all* up to code, your car just won't work the way it did when you first brought it home.

The problem is very similar to the one you might be facing with your brain. You need to have all the elements in place for your brain to work the way it was designed to. Nutrition, exercise, sleep, circadian rhythms, mental challenges, stress release, meaning, and purpose—all of these must be at optimal levels for your brain to function optimally, too. Without even one of these elements, you'll notice a drop in function. Without two, you'll start to feel foggy. And without several, you're likely to feel scattered, unfocused, anxious, depressed, and just "not yourself."

In the next three weeks, through the Brain Fog Fix Program, we're going to get your life back on course by removing the blocks that keep you stuck and giving your brain the materials it needs to heal. The program is set up with each week focusing on one area that affects your brain health: mood, energy, and spirit. I refer to each of these short periods as its own revolution. Seven days to change your mood, seven days to change your energy, and seven days to change your spirit. Here is a basic overview of what I'll ask you to do in order to clear that fog out of your brain. If you'd like to get started right away, turn to page 171, but you might find the program works better if you have a thorough understanding of *why* we are taking these steps, which is what I cover in the rest of the book.

## Banish Brain Fog in 21 Days

### 7-DAY MOOD REVOLUTION

Use the right foods to go from drained and listless to revitalized and energetic. Use cognitive behavioral strategies to remove mental obstacles from your day.

### 7-DAY ENERGY REVOLUTION

Use sleep, circadian rhythms, exercise, and *neurogenesis* to go from foggy and scattered to alert and sharp.

### 7-DAY SPIRIT REVOLUTION

Connect to something larger than yourself to recommit your life's purpose and rediscover your joy in life.

## RECLAIM YOUR FOCUS, MEMORY, AND JOY

I've dedicated my life to helping people think and feel better. In the thousands of hours I have spent with my patients, I've learned a great deal about what keeps people from achieving the lives they seek—what keeps them settling for lackluster jobs, unsatisfying relationships, and uninspiring personal lives.

I've also learned about what enables people to reclaim their focus, memory, and joy. I know that sometimes you need to make some fundamental changes to lead a more fulfilling life. Sometimes you simply need a shift in perspective, an expansion of your coping skills, or a renewed connection to your own deepest sense of self.

But whatever is or is not working in your life, failing to balance your brain chemistry is likely to throw you off. Rebalancing your brain chemistry will enable you to make better decisions, enjoy your life more, and reconnect to what matters most to you.

I am so excited about this book because I know what an extraordinary difference rebalancing your brain chemistry can make in every aspect of your life. If you implement the incredibly straightforward recommendations in this program, you can say good-bye to depression and anxiety. You can bid farewell to brain fog, forgetfulness, and scatterbrain. You can forget about worrying that the "real you" has somehow vanished, leaving this stressed-out, unfocused, and uninspired shell in its place. Learning how to restore your brain to its optimal function will enable you to think and feel better, and allow you to reclaim the power, joy, and purpose that you might have feared were lost forever.

So let's get started! I can't wait for you to see how thrilling your life becomes when your brain is in terrific shape and you are finally feeling like yourself again.

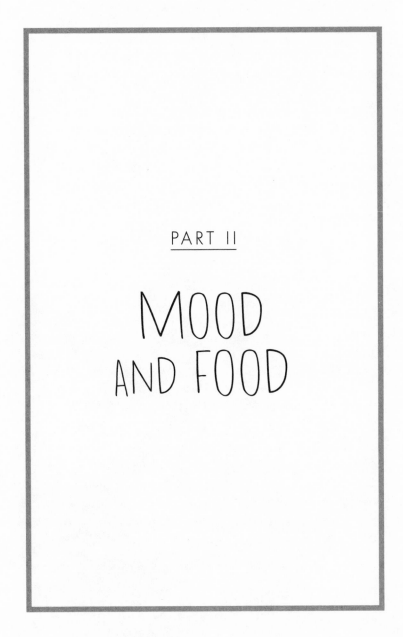

PART II

# MOOD AND FOOD

# CHAPTER 3

# CARBOHYDRATES: HIGHS AND LOWS

Annie, 41, was a single working mom who was 40 to 50 pounds overweight and extremely anxious about it. The first time we met, she rattled off her top three problems: anxiety about not being able to lose weight, anxiety about her inability to find a boyfriend at her current weight, and anxiety about her long-term health and being around to raise her son—which, of course, was related to her weight.

Annie was stuck in a downward spiral. She was anxious, so her serotonin levels were low, which meant she was more likely to crave sugar, flour, and fruit juice. In the short term, she could get temporary relief and a few moments of sweet, sugary bliss, but in the long run, she was facing increasing levels of anxiety and depression.

Annie's primary care doctor had already lectured her on her weight, and she had tried many diets, all to no avail. Like many Americans, Annie had bought into the clever marketing tactics of food companies. She drank bottled store-bought "green juice" and "superfood" pomegranate juice. For breakfast she had "whole-grain" cereal and for snacks she had "natural" chewy granola bars with "no high-fructose corn syrup" and "dark chocolate"–covered almonds instead of chips and candy bars. And she had "reduced-fat" peanut butter on whole-wheat toast instead of white toast and butter in the morning.

Annie had no clue that there were blood sugar–spiking, brain fog–causing, weight gain–inducing villains hidden in just about every single food she was eating. The culprits: sugar and flour. No wonder she was so overweight and depressed!

That store-bought "green juice" was mostly blood sugar–spiking apple juice with a miniscule amount of vegetables and more calories than a full-sugar soda. The same went for the pomegranate juice blend she bought. The first two ingredients: apple and grape juice. Better-for-you-but-more-expensive pomegranate juice was actually the last ingredient listed. The third ingredient listed on her "whole-grain" and "low-fat" cereal: sugar. The second ingredient on these "natural" granola bars: brown sugar. The second ingredient on the "dark chocolate"–covered almonds: sugar. Reduced-fat peanut butter's first two ingredients: corn syrup solids and sugar. Her "whole-wheat" toast contained whole-wheat flour and high-fructose corn syrup, had almost no fiber, and had the same glycemic index as most white bread.

There's nothing wrong with having a little flour or sugar from time to time. But if you're like Annie and most other Americans, you're eating one of these blood sugar–spiking foods every day, at almost every meal and snack—and you may not realize how these ingredients are affecting the way you think and feel.

## BLOOD SUGAR AND THE BRAIN

Blood sugar has a huge bearing on our brain chemistry, and our diets can greatly affect our brains—along with our memories, moods, and concentration levels—for better or worse. The foods we eat can either produce steady, sustaining levels of blood sugar, or they can induce sugar rushes and crashes, which in turn can leave us feeling foggy, listless, anxious, and depressed.

The constant highs and lows that many of us experience aren't just making us fat; they're fundamentally disrupting our brain chemistry. Even worse, our bad dietary and lifestyle habits are setting us up for a future risk of dementia, which has been correlated with perennially high blood-sugar levels.

Most of us understand that overeating or eating the wrong foods contributes to weight gain and a whole host of related health problems like obesity and cardiovascular disease. But it's only recently become clear that these same habits can also lead to depression, serious brain fog or, much worse, dementia or Alzheimer's disease. While researchers don't yet fully understand the precise mechanisms of this relationship, a recent groundbreaking study has linked an "inflammatory dietary pattern" (i.e., foods that cause certain parts of the body to become inflamed) to depression.[1] And the damage doesn't stop there. Research also shows that depression can trigger a cascade of other harmful changes to the brain that can ultimately lead to dementia.[2]

The bottom line is that eating anti-inflammatory foods can actually improve your mood and sharpen your brain, while eating pro-inflammatory foods can do the exact opposite. Increasing the amount of anti-inflammatory foods in your diet may also help to prevent a condition known as leaky brain, in which pro-inflammatory molecules can cross the blood-brain barrier, causing all sorts of problems. (For a more thorough description of the leaky-brain phenomenon, see page 108.) And in the short term, anti-inflammatory foods can counteract some of the inflammatory effects that may be affecting your brain if you are overweight.

## INSULIN AND ALZHEIMER'S

I can't emphasize enough that our diets affect not only how we look but how our brains function. Increased blood sugar can lead to type 2 diabetes, which in turn has been linked to what scientists have over the last decade dubbed "type 3 diabetes": Alzheimer's disease.

Here's how it works. We all need insulin to function: it delivers the blood sugar, or glucose, that cells use for energy. But when we get *too much* glucose and, therefore, insulin—as do many of us who live on high-glycemic-index carbohydrates (cookies, candy, pasta, bread; yes, even whole-wheat bread and gluten-free pizza crust)—our bodies eventually store the excess as fat.

---

## What Is It? Glycemic Index

The glycemic index gives an approximate measure of how much a carbohydrate in a food raises your body's blood-glucose level. A high-glycemic-index (GI) food will raise your glucose level a great deal; a low-GI food will not. Beans, small seeds, and strawberries are examples of low-GI foods, with a ranking below 55. Medium-GI foods like basmati rice and bananas have a ranking between 56 and 69. High-GI foods, the ones so pervasive in our diet, have a GI of more than 70. White bread, white rice, pasta, cookies, candy, cake, and even most whole-wheat bread are all examples of high-GI foods.

---

The more refined carbohydrates we eat, the less our bodies respond to the constant barrage of insulin they create, a condition known as "insulin resistance." That's when type 2 diabetes can develop. Given the contemporary American diet of fast food and prepackaged snacks, it's no wonder that diagnoses of this disease—which, unlike type 1 diabetes, is environmentally caused—have tripled in the U.S. in the past 40 years.[3] Almost one-third of Americans already have diabetes or prediabetes. Just think for a second about how scary that is.

But maybe you're saying, okay, fine, so the worst-case scenario is that I have to learn how to give myself one of those insulin shots, right? Well, not exactly. Unfortunately, these statistics also have a direct bearing on how our brains work. Over the past decade, scientists and researchers have found more and more evidence that insulin resistance acutely affects the brain, which is the reason for Alzheimer's "type 3 diabetes" moniker.

The association between insulin resistance and decreased brain function has long been evident to researchers. One long-term Japanese study found that subjects with diabetes were at a 75 percent increased risk of developing Alzheimer's within 15 years—and 1.75

times more likely to develop dementia—than participants with normal blood-sugar levels. Subjects with impaired glucose tolerance, who might be classified as prediabetic, were 35 percent more likely to develop dementia.[4]

Another study that examined the memory and mental function of 2,300 women between 70 and 78 years old found that women without diabetes were more than twice as likely to score better than those with diabetes. And the longer a woman had diabetes, the more likely she would score poorly on the tests.[5]

Even the physical appearance of diabetes and Alzheimer's are similar, as suggested by one recent study that showed that the plaque deposits in the pancreas in patients with type 2 diabetes resembled the plaque deposits in the brain in patients with Alzheimer's.[6] This suggests that when your blood sugar spikes too often, it wreaks the same havoc in your brain as it does in your body. This means that every time you overindulge in too many unhealthy carbs, you're putting yourself at risk of not being able to remember who your significant other or children are later in life.

Yet another study that showed that *even people without diabetes* who had high blood sugar performed worse on memory tests. What's more, the same study found that people with higher blood-sugar levels had a shrunken hippocampus, which is the part of the brain involved in learning.[7] And you don't have to be downing sodas every hour to be vulnerable: even having moderately above-average blood sugar is associated with decreased brain volume later in life.[8] Another groundbreaking 2013 study of 2,000 people showed participants with higher blood-glucose levels to be at greater risk of developing dementia.[9]

The list goes on and on: obesity without diabetes has been associated with brain impairment, and the authors of still another study found a connection between dementia and not just diabetes but hypertension, or high blood pressure, as well.[10]

Even as wide-ranging research has borne out this troubling connection, scientists have struggled to explain why patients with diabetes and other blood-sugar disorders seem to be at higher risk for cognitive decline. From this outpouring of recent evidence, they've begun to conclude not that diabetes *causes* Alzheimer's, but rather that these two ostensibly unrelated conditions have the exact same root: the environment, in the form of diets that interfere with our bodies' natural response to insulin.

Is it any wonder that as diagnoses of diabetes increase, so do diagnoses of Alzheimer's? Approximately 44 million people were living with dementia in 2013. But the prediction for future cases was 17 percent higher than previous reports. By 2030, that number will have grown to 76 million, and by 2050 to 115 million.[11]

These figures should serve as a real wake-up call: the time has come for us to safeguard both our bodies and our brains from these ravaging conditions. One of the most effective ways to minimize your risk of being among the almost 50 percent of people with Alzheimer's disease or another form of dementia by age 85 is to pay closer attention to your diet.


## HOW FOODS AFFECT OUR BRAINS

Here's a statistic that just blew me away when I first came across it: 95 percent of seniors, as well as most women of childbearing age, are not getting the right amount of *folate,* a type of vitamin B that's essential to the brain. Another B vitamin—vitamin B12—is also critical to brain health, and most of us are deficient in that, too. Many patients diagnosed with Alzheimer's have low levels of vitamin B12, and as many as 30 percent of patients hospitalized for depression are vitamin B12–deficient. Without enough vitamin B, our brains can't make the chemicals we need for mood, brain function, and healthy sleep. It's one of the many dopamine and serotonin cofactors: vitamins your brain needs to convert the amino acids in your diet into feel-good neurochemicals. By not getting the right amounts of vitamin B in your diet—or folate, or vitamin D, or EPA, or DHA, or tryptophan, or tyrosine—you are basically *guaranteeing* that your brain chemistry will be imbalanced and that you will feel anxious, stressed out, uninspired, and depressed, probably with some sleep problems thrown in.

And vitamin B is just *one* of many possible examples! There are several key nutrients that your brain needs to function properly—and if you don't know what they are, chances are you are not getting enough of them.

To complicate matters further, nutrition is just one piece of the puzzle. Your brain also needs exercise, sleep at appropriate intervals, both downtime and stimulation, the chance to continually learn and grow, and sources of meaning and inspiration. Take away any one of these vital factors and your brain chemistry goes out of whack. You think badly and feel worse . . . and you probably don't even know why.

Now perhaps you're beginning to understand that changing how you eat doesn't just make shopping for jeans a whole lot more fun; it can also stabilize your moods and ensure that your brain stays healthy for decades to come. Americans must grapple with these issues more with each passing decade, not just because of our epidemic diabetes rates but because we're living longer than ever. Our increased longevity is in itself a wonderful development—but it means that we must take concrete steps to reduce our long-term risk of cognitive decline and dementia.

Here's roughly how the brain-blood sugar connection works.

The cells in our brain require *twice* as much energy as the cells in the rest of our body. And carbohydrates are the preferred source of energy for our brain. That's why when you're feeling foggy or tired, your tendency might be to reach for something sweet or starchy like chips or a candy bar to revive. That high-glucose food gives you an immediate rush. For a while, your brain has the energy it so desperately needs, and you feel clear, focused, and motivated.

It turns out that our brains need energy boosts while we're concentrating or working, just like our bodies need water and food after a prolonged bout of exercise.[12] Carbs provide that boost to body and brain alike, but *which* carbs is the key question: high GI or low? One study showed that older adults fed a breakfast of mashed potatoes and juice performed 25 percent better in memory tests 20 minutes later than adults who were fed only water.[13]

But while these high-GI foods might help your memory in the short term (and are certainly better than having no food at all), over time they can contribute to insulin resistance. Any too intense infusion of carbs can spike blood-glucose levels, which in turn activates adrenaline. This can cause hyperactivity in children—and in adults, too!—but there are even more serious consequences as well, as we've seen from the alarming link between high blood-sugar levels and decreased brain function.

And—this is crucial—brain cells can't store glucose. That blood-sugar spike inevitably leads to a crash, leaving your poor brain more starved for energy than ever. You feel even foggier and more forgetful than before—and you're even more tempted to reach for either more sweets or some caffeine. So when you think you're feeding your brain, you might just be setting it up for a fall.

High-GI carbs like those in white potatoes and fruit juice act a bit like cocaine on your brain: a spike, followed by a crash. Since carbs are vital to our health, we need to focus our attention on getting the ones that give us the sustainable, slow-burning energy our brains need.

## WHAT TO DO ABOUT IT

The natural response to this news is to say: okay, no problem. If spiking my blood sugar causes weight gain and dementia, then I'll just switch to Diet Coke! While many Americans have taken this path in recent years, there's plenty of evidence out there that shows substituting artificial sweeteners is *not* an effective solution, particularly where your brain is concerned.

In a study of over 2,000 people, the diet-soda drinkers were more likely to be depressed than even the regular-soda or full-sugar-punch drinkers. Recent research sheds some light on this link: artificial sweeteners, it turns out, can disrupt the levels of good bacteria in the gut. This is relevant to your brain because maintaining healthy levels of bacteria in the gut has been linked to both mood and cognition. Remember: the vast majority of the serotonin in your body is manufactured in your gut. So by disrupting your belly, you're disrupting the chemicals in your brain, a cycle that can have seriously mood-altering consequences. If you really need a sweetener, do yourself a favor and switch from Splenda to natural stevia.

▶ **EXPERT'S TIP:** If you prefer coffee or tea to these drinks, that's fantastic—but watch what you add to these beverages. If you're in the habit of putting milk and some form of sweetener in your tea of coffee, you should be aware that milk itself is already a source of sugar, so by adding both, you are *double* spiking your blood sugar. For more on coffee and tea, see pages 68 to 69.

I can't emphasize enough the importance of breaking your dependence on artificial sweeteners if you're trying to fight brain fog. They might save you a few calories, but they aren't giving your brain the nutrients it requires for optimum performance. The real answer is a slow and steady supply of glucose, which we get from the carbohydrates in our diet. Does that mean you need to eat potatoes at every meal? Absolutely not, because foods you probably don't think of as "carbs" are already giving you carbs. Many foods you may think of as protein sources have carbs. Beans have carbs. And again, every time you drink milk, you're getting some carbs in addition to protein and fat.

The key to regulating your brain chemistry—and to keeping dementia at bay—is to limit your intake of carbs, or to replace the high-GI carbohydrates that trigger blood-sugar spikes (and subsequent crashes) with more complex carbohydrates. The first step is to start cutting back on carbs in the form of flour and sugar, which the vast majority of Americans consume in excess.

These high-GI carbohydrates are everywhere, and they've made their way into even the most innocent-seeming foods: companies have added sugars to fats like salad dressing, and flour to meats in the form of breading and sugar-laden sauces, and sugar in traditionally sugarless drinks like coffee. (Of course, it doesn't help that processed carbohydrates are the most profitable for food companies, which is one big reason they're also the most readily available.) By cutting back dramatically on flour and sugar, you will not only reduce blood-sugar spikes, but you'll also increase the amount of anti-inflammatory foods in your diet as you replace them with more vegetables, beans, and fish.

Swapping flour- and sugar-loaded foods for healthier alternatives is easier than you might think. Try sprouted, flourless bread instead of your favorite white (or even whole-wheat) bread. Instead of white rice or pasta, try mixing your veggies with quinoa or sprouted barley. Instead of regular white pasta, try zucchini noodles or shirataki noodles (see page 178). Instead of macaroni salad, try an organic egg or chickpea salad.

These "swaps" are better for two reasons. First, they significantly bring down the glycemic load of your food: white and even most whole-wheat breads have a glycemic index in the 70s, whereas sprouted bread has a glycemic index in the 30s. Instead of rice, try sprouted barley. With just one simple substitution, you'll have reduced your blood-sugar spikes by at least half—and you'll also think and feel better in the process. Making these easy substitutions is also great for weight loss.

Second, slow-burning carbohydrates contain amino acids like tryptophan, which is a precursor to serotonin. These foods also allow tryptophan to "get in" the brain. The blood-brain barrier is the gatekeeper that allows nutrients you need in while keeping toxins out to protect your most precious organ. This process is facilitated by what's known as transporters that recognize tryptophan and other amino acids. When tryptophan lingers—through the help of a slow-burning carb—more of this mood-boosting amino acid gets into the brain, and you feel better as a result.

Why exactly is this the case? When we don't get enough tryptophan (along with the cofactors it needs, such as folate, which I explain on pages 64 to 65), our brains just aren't able to produce the serotonin that soothes anxiety and boosts mood. (Note to vegetarians: many vegetarians are tryptophan deficient, so you need to go out of your way to make sure that you get enough of this important amino acid. Sesame seeds, sunflower seeds, and bananas are great sources.)

When you aren't making enough serotonin, guess what you crave: carbs! Processed carbohydrates release big doses of serotonin in the brain in the same way that cocaine releases big doses of dopamine. If your brain isn't getting enough serotonin through healthy food, you will end up self-medicating with unhealthy food to achieve that same state. Luckily, it's easy to swap out the brain-endangering carbs with healthy, sustaining ones.

## ACTION PLAN: BLOOD-SUGAR SWAPS

Now that you know that blood-sugar spikes can cause brain fog and even lead to dementia, I am going to teach you how to introduce a wide variety of foods into your diet that will give you steady, small amounts of complex carbohydrates—like transitioning from processed fruit juice to whole fruit or veggie juice. After jumping into the 7-Day Mood Revolution, you'll soon make these healthier alternatives a normal part of your everyday diet . . . and you'll feel much better as a consequence.

---

### The 80/20 Rule

Once you've completed the 7-Day Mood Revolution, you will start to follow my 80/20 rule, meaning that 80 percent of the time, you eat these brain-healthy foods, and the other 20 percent of the time, you can let loose a bit (but within reason!). Because yes, I do understand that there are certain special occasions—from your vacation to Italy to Super Bowl Sunday—when you will just want to down that plate of pasta or a little too much pizza. An occasional indulgence is perfectly all right!

---

Protecting your blood sugar is as good for your brain as it is for your body. Here are some simple additions to your diet that can minimize blood-sugar spikes. You should be eating these foods regularly whether you embark on my 21-day program or not:

#1: *Cinnamon.* Sprinkle cinnamon in your coffee instead of a packet of sugar. By making this change, you'll prevent a brain-fogging blood-sugar spike. Cinnamon also has anti-inflammatory and antioxidant effects, whereas sugar creates inflammation.

#2: *Raw or slightly cooked vegetables.* The more you cook a vegetable, the more you may compromise the blood sugar–blocking capabilities of the fiber it contains. This fiber can minimize some of the blood-sugar spikes created by carbs, especially when you eat the vegetable before the carb.

#3: *Vinegar.* Vinegar has been shown to keep blood-sugar levels in check by preventing some of the starch in bread or pasta from turning into sugar. You'll effortlessly lower your blood sugar by switching from store-bought salad dressings that often contain sugar to a simple blend of vinegar and olive oil.

#4: *Tea.* Tea may reduce the amount of glucose absorbed by the intestine, which reduces blood-sugar spikes. So drink a glass of unsweetened, black iced tea at lunch. One study showed black tea did this better than other types of tea. White tea was second best at preventing blood-sugar spikes and also contains very little caffeine, which makes it a great choice to accompany dinner at night.[14]

#5: *Red wine.* As we'll see later in this section, for those without a history of alcoholism or problem drinking, a glass of red wine with dinner may lessen blood-sugar spikes by preventing intestinal glucose absorption and reducing your liver's production of glucose. One study found that red wine may be more effective at blocking glucose absorption than white wine.[15]

# Simple Swaps

Here are some simple swaps and switches to help reduce blood-sugar spikes:

- Cut the pasta in half and sub zucchini or spaghetti squash noodles for half. You can use a vegetable peeler.

- When you do cook pasta, make it al dente. Overcooking pasta increases its glycemic index, so set the timer for a minute or two below the suggested cooking time.

- When you're making pasta, use half as much pasta and add broccoli or cauliflower. When I make my favorite childhood treat, macaroni and cheese, I throw out half the pasta and add bulk with broccoli and cauliflower. (Of course, I also use organic milk and butter.)

- At Subway, ask for your bread to be "shelled out" to cut your carbs in half. While you're at it, ask for low-glycemic veggies like spinach, tomatoes, olives, and green peppers. Load up on low-GI dressings like vinegar and mustard. Or when you get your sandwich, just eat half of the bread.

- When ordering pizza, ditch the deep dish or traditional for thin crust. Instead of eating four slices for dinner, eat a big salad with vinegar and olive oil first and then just one or two slices of pizza.

CHAPTER 4

# Dietary Fats: The Good, the Bad, and the Ugly

Jeremy was a high-strung entrepreneur in his early 50s. He was recently divorced and struggling with work stress, health issues, and the guilt that came with only getting to see his kids on weekends.

With my help, Jeremy started to use some cognitive behavioral strategies (outlined on pages 171 through 193 in the Brain Fog Fix Program) to improve his outlook. He also started to tweak his diet—with results that he admitted astonished him.

You see, Jeremy *thought* he was eating the right foods. He bought low-fat balsamic vinaigrette for salad dressing, ate lots of grilled chicken, forced down a chia-seed drink once a week, and had low-fat tuna salad on wheat bread a few times a month.

But Jeremy's "healthy" diet—particularly his choice of fats—represented an all-too-common pitfall in the American diet: he ate far too many omega-6s and not enough omega-3s.

Jeremy's low-fat, low-calorie balsamic vinaigrette, made by a big food company, contained *no* olive oil at all. Instead, his brand of choice used cheap-for-them, bad-for-you soybean oil. His go-to lunch of non-organic grilled chicken was giving him too many pro-inflammatory omega-6s as well. The chia-seed drink helped some, but because his body had to convert the omega-3 alpha-linolenic acid (ALA) into the "think better" omega-3 docosahexaenoic acid (DHA) and the "feel better" omega-3 eicosapentaenoic acid (EPA), he wasn't getting nearly enough of the truly beneficial ingredients. And his occasional tuna salad wasn't giving him enough omega-3 DHA, either. What's worse, the albacore contained too much mercury, and his favorite low-fat mayo also used soybean instead of olive oil. Even a food he never thought contained oils—wheat bread—contained harmful hydrogenated oils!

As I helped Jeremy change his diet, his mood began to improve, and he found that he was having an easier time navigating his difficult life transition. Jeremy was pleasantly surprised that his new diet of anti-inflammatory, healthier fats actually tasted better. He ditched "light" salad dressing for real olive oil and balsamic vinegar. These good fats are more filling than low-calorie, sugar-laden dressings, so he also noticed that by eating better, he felt more satisfied than he had when he used to choose the "diet" food.

Of course, food was just a one of the many reasons Jeremy started to think and feel better. He also worked on healing his relationship with his kids and forgiving himself for his marriage not working out. By focusing on what he *could* control in his life, he had an easier time accepting what he couldn't.

## FATS: NOT ALL CREATED EQUAL

The high-sugar, low-fiber processed carbohydrates that spike your blood sugar and set you up for brain fog and depression are just one piece of the nutritional puzzle. You must also take into account fats, which can leave you thinking and feeling a whole lot better—or worse.

Eating the healthiest fats—which include monounsaturated fats like olive oil and the anti-inflammatory, high omega-3 fat found in seafood—can play a big role in preserving the health of your brain. (They're also particularly vital to developing brains. In 2014, the FDA revised its recommendation for pregnant women and young children, advising they eat between two and three servings of low-mercury seafood a week.) Everyone, regardless of age, should be eating healthy fats regularly. One study showed people who consumed the healthiest fats were 42 percent less likely to experience cognitive impairment![1]

So toss out the old notion that fat is the enemy. It is actually one of the most important things you can eat to improve the health of your brain, and most of us should probably be eating *more*, not less, of the right kinds of fats. Unfortunately, it can be extremely difficult to figure out which are the good fats and which are the bad ones just from glancing at a food label. There tends to be some crucial information missing, like how much of the fat is anti-inflammatory omega-3s and how much is pro-inflammatory omega-6s. Let's walk through this basic information that's so crucial for the long-term health of our brains.

## WHY YOU NEED OMEGA-3S

The absolute best fats for your brain are omega-3 fatty acids, which help prevent inflammation—the key, we now know, to preserving cognitive function and warding off depression, stress, and anxiety. Omega-3s can lower our risk of developing chronic diseases like heart disease and arthritis, and they can even make it hard for cancer cells to survive.[2] They play an important role in both cognition and behavior, and they're the building blocks for important hormones that govern immune function and cell growth.

These omega-3 fatty acids are considered essential, which means the body needs them but cannot make them on its own. We can get them *only* through food, and that's why it's so important to go out of our way to incorporate these amazing fats into our diets as frequently as possible.

Several different types of omega-3s govern the health of our brains. The most important ones are DHA, which is mainly associated with cognition, and EPA, which is associated primarily with mood. We need both of these fatty acids for optimum brain health, but we're not getting nearly enough of either! Among the top ten preventable causes of death in the U.S. are smoking, obesity, physical inactivity, and . . . a lack of omega-3s.[3] Like smoking and overeating, a lack of omega-3s can lead to diseases that ultimately result in death.

It's important to understand the three different types of omega-3s. Omega-3s react with the body in different ways, and they carry out distinct functions in the brain.

ALA is a vegetarian source of omega-3s. You can get it from "omega-3 enriched" pasta, flaxseeds, walnuts, and canola oil. The problem is that your body has to convert ALA into DHA and EPA to get the biggest benefits, and your body is not very good at this conversion, especially if you're a man. ALA has still been shown to decrease inflammation, but it's far more efficient to go straight to the main source of EPAs and DHAs in seafood.[4] Vegans—many of whom are deficient in DHA—can get this nutrient from a supplement that uses algae instead of fish oil.

## Converting ALA

Conversion rates for healthy young men:

- 8 percent of the ALA is converted into EPA
- 0 to 4 percent of the ALA is converted into DHA

Conversion rates for healthy young women:

- 21 percent of the ALA is converted into EPA
- 9 percent of the ALA is converted in DHA

Women might get twice the DHA and EPA as men because of their higher estrogen levels, which is helpful during pregnancy, when estrogen soars and the baby gets lots of DHA that is essential for brain development. But older women who are going through or have been through menopause have much lower estrogen levels, and they need to make a real effort to get EPA and DHA straight from the source, no conversion required.

**DHA,** your brain's "think better" omega-3, is found mostly in fish, seaweed, and DHA-enriched milk. Associated with cognition, DHA can improve IQ scores and support neurogenesis. DHA is particularly critical to the developing brain—that's why pregnant moms and kids need so much of it. It is also important for preventing brain fog, dementia, and Alzheimer's disease. In fact, one large-scale study showed that the people with the highest levels of DHA, who ate three servings of fish a week, were 47 percent less likely to develop dementia and 39 percent less likely to develop Alzheimer's than those with lower levels of DHA.[5]

**EPA** is your brain's "feel better" omega-3, which, like DHA, you can get mostly through seafood. (Most seafood has a little more DHA than EPA, but a few types have more EPA than DHA.) People with low levels of omega-3s are more likely to be depressed and even diagnosed with ADHD.[6] Boosting the brain's EPA levels can do wonders for improving mood, preventing depression, and soothing anxiety. One study showed a link between people who ate a lot of fish and good mood.[7] Another even larger study found that those taking an omega-3 fish oil supplement were about 30 percent less likely to exhibit depressive symptoms than those not taking one.[8] Supplementing with fish oils that have a high EPA to DHA ratio has been shown to lead to significant reductions in both depressive symptoms and anxiety: a wonderful study of stressed-out medical students subject to frequent exams showed that omega-3 supplementation resulted in a 20 percent reduction in anxiety symptoms while simultaneously decreasing inflammation.[9]

**EXPERT'S TIP: Beating the Blues with EPA:** If you struggle with depression or anxiety, talk to your primary care physician or psychiatrist to see if adding a high-EPA omega-3 supplement might help. Most omega-3 supplements have a near 1:1 ratio of EPA to DHA, but the ratio with the most data supporting mood improvement is approximately 7:1 EPA to DHA. The two brands that contain this ratio are OM3

Emotional Balance and Country Life Omega-3 Mood, both of which provide approximately 1,000 mg of EPA and just 150 mg of DHA. Although further research is necessary, formulas containing just EPA with no DHA could be even more effective for improving mood. Omegavia EPA 500 is a brand with all EPA. For people with depression or anxiety, these high-EPA supplements can be a very effective alternative—or have a helpful additive effect—to prescription medications like Prozac and Xanax. And unlike most prescription medications, which have many side effects, fish oil comes with a host of health benefits.

## GETTING THE RATIO RIGHT

Most people think of omega-3s like they do vitamin C or calcium: just get the recommended daily value and you're good. But it's not *just* getting enough omega-3s that counts; you also have to minimize your omega-6s, which can promote inflammation and lead to some serious health problems. Like omega-3s, omega-6s are essential, which means your body doesn't produce them on its own; you need to get them in the food you eat.

The problem is that modern diets contain *far* too many omega-6s, especially in comparison to omega-3s. Omega-6s are found in a wide range of processed foods and refined vegetable oils, including the soybean oil that lurks in just about every single packaged food out there.

Omega-3s and 6s have complementary functions in the body and brain: omega-3s decrease inflammation whereas omega-6s promote inflammation. Humans likely evolved on a diet that was a 1:1 ratio of these essential fatty acids.

Recently, however—thanks to factory-farmed animal products, the world takeover of processed snack foods, and a decrease in fish intake—this ratio has skewed strongly in favor of omega-6s. The ideal omega-6 to omega-3 ratio should be about 2 to 1, but most Americans now get 10 to 25 times more omega-6s than omega-3s. This imbalance can lead to more inflammation. More depression. More anxiety. More brain fog.

Bringing this ratio back into balance is an important step in thinking and feeling better.

## UPPING YOUR OMEGA-3S

So how do you get more omega-3s into your diet? The short answer: fish, fish, and more fish. There's probably *nothing* more beneficial to the brain than eating the right kind of seafood. One study that followed hundreds of men over a decade demonstrated that men who did not eat fish experienced *four times* more cognitive decline than those who ate fish regularly, and the DHA in fish has been shown to fight the plaques that are the hallmark of Alzheimer's disease.[10]

> **EXPERT'S TIP:** Taking a supplement is fine, but it's only half the battle. To reap the greatest health benefits, you should be regularly eating actual fish as well. That's because there are cofactors (for an explanation, see pages 66 to 67) in fish like selenium, zinc, and iron that help your body maximize the benefits of omega-3s. Some of these nutrients have their own brain-protective benefits. Selenium, for example, has been shown to improve both cognition and mood and may also help prevent postpartum depression.[11] Low selenium levels have also been linked with cognitive decline.[12]

But not all fish are created equal. Some can be deceptively high in omega-6s. Many farm-raised fish, for example—particularly tilapia, which is everywhere these days—are fed foods high in omega-6s, so they won't deliver the infusion of omega-3s that our brains so desperately need.[13]

Mercury pollution is another factor to consider when choosing fish, since mercury toxicity has been linked to memory loss and depression.[14] The developing brain is especially sensitive to mercury exposure: mothers with more mercury in their system had children with lower cognitive scores.[15] But while our primary exposure to mercury is through fish, we shouldn't avoid fish, which truly is one of the brain-healthiest foods out there. Proof: mothers who ate more fish—but less mercury—had infants with *better* cognition.[16]

The key is to choose the fish with the highest concentration of omega-3s and the lowest content of toxins. A general rule of thumb is to favor wild-caught over farm-raised fish. And while they don't pack quite the omega-3 punch of salmon or sardines, shrimp and scallops give you a moderate dose of omega-3, and they're fairly low in toxins.[17]

**EXPERT'S TIP:** The fish-loving Japanese don't worry much about mercury for the simple reason that they often drink tea with their fish. Black coffee and green or black tea can reduce your mercury exposure by over 50 percent. This is especially important when you eat sushi, as uncooked fish will expose you to more mercury than cooked fish.[18]

To simplify matters, the Monterey Bay Aquarium teamed up with the Harvard School of Public Health and the Environmental Defense Fund to come up with a fairly short list of go-to fish that are high in omega-3s, low in pollutants like mercury and PCBs, and sustainably caught.

Here are the fish you want to make the focus of your diet:

- Albacore tuna, troll or pole caught, fresh or canned, U.S. or British Columbia
- Arctic char, farmed
- Barramundi, farmed, U.S.
- Coho salmon, farmed, U.S.
- Dungeness crab, wild, California, Oregon, or Washington
- Longfin squid, wild, Atlantic
- Mussels, farmed

- Oysters, farmed
- Pacific sardines, wild
- Pink shrimp, wild, Oregon
- Rainbow trout, farmed
- Salmon, wild, Alaska
- Spot prawns, wild, British Columbia

The list of fish you are better off avoiding is, unfortunately, just as long:

- Canned light tuna
- Canned albacore tuna
  (except those labeled troll or pole caught)
- Tuna steaks
- Lobster
- Carp
- Flatfish
- Bass
- Perch
- Haddock
- Hake
- Snapper
- Halibut
- Mackerel
- Roughy
- Sea bass
- Shark
- Swordfish
- Tilapia
- Tilefish

In addition to their toxin content, many of these fish contain far fewer of the "think and feel better" omega-3s than the choices in the first list.

> **EXPERT'S TIP**: If all of this information is making your head spin, I recommend the amazing app and downloadable regional guides available at seafoodwatch.org. For specific buying tips, please see pages 181 to 183 in Part VI.

## ANOTHER HEALTHY SOURCE OF FAT: OLIVE OIL

As omega-3s prove, fat is by no means inherently bad for you, and neither is cholesterol. In fact, some studies have shown that for both men and women, cholesterol levels that are too low have been linked to depressive symptoms.[19] It's not just the cholesterol level itself but also the *type* of cholesterol that's important. Bad cholesterol, the kind found in saturated fats and trans fats, has been linked to amyloid plaque in the brain—the hallmark of Alzheimer's. The worst type of cholesterol is oxysterol, the one found in fried foods and partially hydrogenated oils.

It's important to cut back on unhealthy saturated fats and get more monounsaturated fats, which can lower LDL cholesterol—the "bad" cholesterol—without lowering HDL cholesterol, the "good" one. The best source of monounsaturated fat in the diet: olive oil.

Extra virgin olive oil (for salad dressings) and olive oil (for cooking, since virgin oil isn't as stable at high temperatures) are your best bets for thinking and feeling better. Olive oil is a potent source of a variety of anti-inflammatory compounds including polyphenols, which may prevent Alzheimer's disease and depression; it also contains high levels of oleic acid, which is a healthy, monounsaturated omega-9 oil. (Omega-9s are monounsaturated fats that are great for you, but unlike omega-3s and 6s, your body can produce them, so they're not considered essential.)

To maximize the olive oil in your diet, you should be spraying olive oil on your (toasted flourless) bread at breakfast, adding a tablespoon of olive oil to your salad at lunch, *and* cooking your wild salmon in olive oil at dinner. (See pages 173 to 184 for tips on where to get the healthiest foods.) It's just an incredible ingredient for your brain.

A large-scale study found that people who used olive oil for both cooking *and* dressing had the best cognitive function as they aged, even compared to those who just used it for one or the other.[20] This "intensive" use of olive oil is also associated with a 41 percent decreased risk of stroke.[21] Olive oil consumption—in combination with fish and vegetables—has been linked to a reduced risk of mild cognitive impairment, including impairment that can progress to Alzheimer's disease.[22]

Olive oil can help you feel better as well. The olive oil–rich Mediterranean diet has been shown to protect against depression.[23] People who eat a diet high in trans fats have a 48 percent increased risk of depression compared to those who eat a diet high in healthy fats like olive oil, nuts, and fish.[24]

If you're out of olive oil, canola oil is an okay second choice since its fat composition is close to that of olive oil. Soybean oil, by contrast, is an ingredient you should try to minimize or eliminate in your diet, since you're already ingesting a great deal of it whether you know it or not. Chances are, if you have any store-bought dressings, mayonnaise, or spaghetti sauce in your pantry, a good many of them have soybean oil in them. Go read the ingredients on the back of the bottles—see what I mean? This is a problem because soybean oil has more polyunsaturated fat than monounsaturated fat, and it's a leading source of omega-6s in the American diet. Cutting back on it will go a long way toward restoring the optimal omega-3 to omega-6 ratio in your diet.

For specific shopping recommendations, please turn to pages 173 to 184 in the 7-Day Mood Revolution. Even if you think you're eating the right fats, you might be amazed how much better you will feel by making some incredibly simple swaps—like eliminating soybean oil in favor of olive, or having a wild salmon salad sandwich instead of your usual tuna.

# CHAPTER 5

# Proteins: The Building Blocks of the Body—and Brain

Caitlyn was a svelte woman in her early 30s who worked in the fashion industry. She lived what she thought was a very healthy lifestyle. Like many American women, she had bought into the hype of the high-protein weight management trend in food marketing, which includes an emphasis on cutting out high-fat and carb-heavy foods. Her diet consisted mostly of protein shakes with skim milk, high-protein soy products, eggs, and grilled chicken salads. She came to me because she'd been feeling irritable and anxious—and she couldn't figure out why. She wanted to *feel* good in addition to *looking* good.

While a diet high in protein can be part of a healthy diet, it's important to eat *high-quality* protein if you want to improve mood. The tricky part is that omega-3 and omega-6 content isn't listed on nutritional labels, and getting enough omega-3s is vital to reducing inflammation, anxiety, and depression. So while a grilled chicken breast that's not organic may help you lose weight, it's also high in omega-6s and low in omega-3s. Organic chicken breast, wild salmon, and walnuts are better choices that help you feel better while simultaneously preventing weight gain.

So Caitlyn and I focused on changing her diet. One of the hardest changes I asked her to make was to switch from fat-free, conventional skim milk to low-fat organic milk. This would help her get more anxiety-reducing omega-3s. And while it contains more calories than skim milk, it would also help her feel fuller longer. This simple swap would also help her body absorb fat-soluble vitamin D (among other vitamins), which would improve her energy levels.

She also looked at the other proteins she was eating in order to switch to organic animal products and clean seafood, which provide more feel-good omega-3s and fewer pro-inflammatory omega-6s. She replaced cheap soy burgers with slightly higher-calorie blackbean burgers and even the occasional organic, grass-fed beef burger. Caitlyn also started eating one serving of clean seafood every day. She slowly came to understand that low calorie and low carb don't always mean healthier.

We also added more carbs to Caitlyn's diet, in the form of beans, whole fruits, organic dairy, and healthy grains. These healthy carbohydrates helped boost her serotonin levels, which reduced her anxiety even more. Caitlyn was learning that carbohydrates are not inherently bad just as protein is not inherently good. It's a delicate balancing act that requires us to investigate beyond the numbers on the nutritional label. Bit by bit, Caitlyn began to make small changes in her diet—and she felt far less on edge.

In the end, the changes Caitlyn made in her diet were among many larger changes she made in other parts of her life, which included a newfound meditation practice and making exercise a priority. Before too long, Caitlyn noticed a significant difference in the way she felt. Workdays flew by, and stress, while still present, felt more manageable. With a few simple changes in her diet, Caitlyn felt much more at ease in her daily life.

## PUZZLING OUT PROTEIN

Along with carbohydrates and fats, proteins are the other major component of our diets—though of course all of these categories overlap a great deal. Fish is a source of protein as well as healthy fats, and milk contains both carbohydrates and protein. Because this program is holistic, we will be looking at all of these foods and how they affect our brains and behavior.

As with fats, it can be difficult to figure out the best types of proteins to eat. When it comes to foods like meat, dairy, eggs, and tofu, you won't find the most important information on the nutritional label. These crucial items might be missing:

- The presence of hormones, antibiotics, and pesticides
- The type of feed used and for how much of the lifespan
- The isoflavone content of soy products
- The content of amino acids like tryptophan and tyrosine
- How the food is processed

Let's run through some types of protein and how you can optimize the brain benefits of each.

## SOY

While some natural forms of soy can be healthy, Americans overload on processed products like soy protein isolate, textured soy, vegetable protein, and soy flour: cheap ingredients that food companies use to add protein or enhance texture in all sorts of different foods. This processing can add huge amounts of isoflavones—estrogenlike structures that have been linked to infertility and altered ovarian function in animal studies—to food.[1] Soy protein isolate is of particular concern to vegetarians who regularly eat soy burgers, soy yogurt, and meat substitutes.

**EXPERT'S TIP:** If you're a vegetarian, skip the cheap soy burgers made with nonorganic soy protein; instead get your protein from beans and sprouted grains, or make your own veggie burgers from black beans and chickpeas. You can also look for varieties with soy protein labeled organic or non-GMO.

We already learned in the previous chapter that soybean oil gives us too many omega-6 fats, but that's not the only problem with soy. Nonorganic or non-GMO soy has one of the highest levels of pesticides of any nonorganic food, and if that weren't bad enough, over 90 percent of the soybeans in the U.S. are genetically modified.

The controversy surrounding GMOs—genetically modified organisms—could fill a whole book, so I will say simply that the only thing we *do* know is that we don't know how GMOs will affect human health, including the health of the brain, over the long term. And when it comes to soybeans, GMO versions are generally packed with pesticides. This is because soybeans are genetically modified to be immune to pesticides, so the crops can be sprayed without being killed. Not exactly what you had in mind when you ordered those "healthy" veggie sausages at breakfast this morning, is it?

Nonorganic soy is even more problematic because the vast majority of processed soy relies on hexane extraction. Hexane is a toxic petroleum byproduct. The amount of this neurotoxin that gets into food is not tested for or disclosed in the ingredients since it's just used in the "processing" of the food. But hexane has been shown to cause symptoms such as headache, nausea, and fatigue. If you buy soy products that say USDA organic or 100 percent organic, they won't be processed with hexane, but even products labeled "made with organic ingredients" on the front can include nonorganic soy processed with hexane. For all these reasons, it's safer to stick with soy products labeled organic or non-GMO.

But I'm not saying all soy is bad—not at all! Eaten whole, as nature made it, soy is a complete protein, meaning it contains all the essential amino acids, including tryptophan and tyrosine, which we need to make serotonin and dopamine, respectively. Soy protein itself may actually increase the levels of feel-good serotonin in the brain and improve mood.[2] Soy lecithin may help people deal with stress by decreasing the amount of stress hormone released in tricky situations.[3] Soy might also improve cognition.[4] To reap these benefits, you don't need much soy—just a serving a day.

But what kind of soy should you eat? The very best soy for both vegetarians and nonvegetarians is *fermented soy*, a category that includes tempeh, miso, natto, and tamari, all of which have potent anticancer properties in addition to their brain-boosting ones. Non-fermented soy—which includes all processed soy, like soy protein isolate, and textured vegetable protein—has antinutrient properties that can contribute to depression, weight gain, and fatigue. Fermenting the soy deactivates these harmful processes. While fermented soy like tempeh is the healthiest form of soy, whole soy in the form of tofu and edamame are your next-best choices and are fairly healthy when eaten in moderation.

## Soy Dos and Don'ts: A Recap

1. One serving of a soy food per day may help you think and feel better.

2. Fermented whole soy products like tempeh, miso, and natto are better than processed soy products like soy protein isolate.

3. Tofu and edamame, while not as healthy as fermented soy, are better than processed soy products like soy protein isolate.

4. Organic or non-GMO soy products are better than nonorganic soy products.

## ANIMAL PRODUCTS

When it comes to animal products, I can't emphasize enough the importance of going organic. Like organic fruits and vegetables, organic milk, eggs, dairy, and meat are *far* cleaner and safer than their conventional counterparts—and I would argue well worth the extra money. In fact, choosing organic milk, eggs, dairy, and meat is even more important than choosing organic produce. While both organic produce and animal products are cleaner in general, organic animal products have more brain-healthy, anti-inflammatory omega-3s and fewer omega-6s.

Egg-laying hens and milk-producing cows allowed to roam in open air live in far cleaner conditions than animals sequestered in the disgusting, feces-contaminated cages and pens of conventional factory farms. The pervasive filth can lead to infections, which is one reason factory farms have historically pumped their animals full of antibiotics. This practice has led to bacteria that have become resistant to these drugs in both animals and humans.

### Meat

Let's start with meat. There's a big difference between the saturated fats in the average cheeseburger and those in a lean cut of organic grass-fed beef. Beef labeled organic, grass-fed, free-roaming, or pastured tends to have significantly *more* omega-3s and significantly *fewer* omega-6s. The average conventionally raised beef will have an omega-6 to omega-3 ratio of 7.65 to 1. Grass-fed beef brings the omega-6 content *way down* to about 1.5 to 1, an excellent ratio.[5]

The same goes for other meat. The meat from free-roaming chickens has more omega-3s than that from grain-fed chickens.[6] (But remember: The *type* of omega-3 in animal products, including dairy, meat, and eggs, is primarily ALA. While ALA is good, it doesn't come close to the power of EPA and DHA, which are found mostly in fish.)

Conventional meat might also contain PCBs and dioxins, industrial byproducts that have largely been banned but persist in our environment and may contribute to cancer and neurological problems.[7]

PCBs and dioxins are the result of industrial processes like pesticide production, so grass-fed and organic meat generally contains less of these toxins. Grass-fed meat also tends to be leaner than conventional meats, which can make it less carcinogenic. The types of chemicals that form when the amino acids in meat are exposed to high temperatures have been shown to be carcinogenic.[8]

The leaner the meat you choose, the less you'll be exposed to these risks. Whatever type of meat you're preparing, marinate before you grill, flip it frequently, and eat it medium rare instead of well done. All of these strategies have been shown to help reduce meat's toxicity.

Another deceptively "healthy" variety of conventional meat is processed lunchmeat. While some lunchmeats can be lean, they are almost always made from conventionally raised animals, which means they seldom contain enough of the omega-3s that nourish the brain. Instead, they tend to be high in those pro-inflammatory omega-6s that have been associated with poor mood. If that wasn't enough, a study of 200,000 people revealed those who ate the most processed meats had a 68 percent increased risk of one of the deadliest kinds of cancer—pancreatic cancer—compared to those who ate the least. This likely has to do with the way lunchmeat is processed, so it's generally a good idea to stay away from all processed lunchmeat—even if it's grass-fed meat. People who ate the most red meat also had a significantly increased risk of pancreatic cancer, but not as much as those who ate processed meats. That's yet another compelling reason to reduce meat consumption.

## Dairy

Organic milk is another way to increase the omega-3s (and decrease the omega-6s) in your diet. A large-scale nationwide study of organic versus conventional milk found that the organic variety contained 62 percent more omega-3s and 25 percent fewer omega-6s than conventional. That's a huge difference!

You can enjoy more of these healthy fats by ditching your watery, conventional skim milk, since skimming the fat off also means reducing the omega-3 content. And despite logic that says to cut fat to stay slim, a 2013 study found that children who drink low-fat milk were less likely to be slim than children who drank the full-fat varieties.[9] So instead of skim milk, choose varieties that contain fat—just make sure whatever you get is organic.

Drinking organic dairy will also help correct the all-too-common vitamin D deficiency, which can lead to a depressed mood. Since Vitamin D is fat soluble, it needs to be consumed with fat to be used by the body. And while saturated fat from conventional dairy may be bad for the heart, the conjugated linoleic acid (CLA) found in *organic* dairy offsets the adverse effects—namely heart attacks—of the saturated fat it contains.[10] There's also more CLA in organic and grass-fed beef, which seems to protect your heart from this source of fat as well. In short, our knee-jerk association of the terms *cholesterol* and *saturated fat* applies mostly to conventionally raised meat and dairy.

## Eggs

As with other animal products, organic eggs tend to be far healthier than their conventional counterparts. One recent experiment found that eggs from chickens allowed to roam and eat nutritious grasses have more than double the omega-3s than those fed an industrial diet as well as more vitamins.[11]

With less saturated fat and the CLA that safeguards the heart, organic eggs from free-roaming or pastured chickens that are free to eat nutritious grasses instead of pesticide-laden GMO foods are entirely different from the conventionally grown varieties. But it can be tricky to choose the healthiest eggs at the supermarket—which is exactly the intention of conventional egg producers focused on maximizing profits. Don't be fooled by any of the following terms on egg boxes:

- All natural
- Cage-free
- Vegetarian-fed
- Pasteurized

"Omega-3 fortified" eggs will greatly increase the ratio of omega-3s to omega-6s, but feeding chickens ALA-rich flaxseed doesn't mean you will be eating eggs from chickens that don't eat pesticide-laden grains or aren't treated with hormones.

The words to look for are one or more of the following:

- Organic
- Free-roaming
- Pastured

## ALTERNATE PROTEIN SOURCES: MAKING THE ADJUSTMENT

I'm the first to admit that organic animal products cost more than their conventional counterparts, but there are ways to offset your grocery bill. The most important one—for the health of both your wallet and your brain—is to try cutting the amount of meat, dairy, and eggs you consume in half. Most Americans eat far too many animal products as it is.

You can easily increase your intake of protein from sources like clean fish and sprouted bread, two slices of which have eight grams of protein. Eat just three ounces of wild salmon and two slices of sprouted bread, and you've already consumed 30 grams of protein—more than half of the 45 to 55 grams moderately active people need in a day. Beans are another great protein option, with about 15 grams of protein per serving. They're also one of the richest sources of antioxidants, which can neutralize the effects of damage in your brain and possibly reduce your risk of Alzheimer's and Parkinson's, and they cost a fraction of what you pay for meat.[12] By swapping some of the meat in your diet for beans, you're saving money while boosting antioxidants and reducing inflammation.

Beans also have a favorable omega-3 to -6 ratio. Unlike factory-farmed chicken, some high-protein beans have more omega-3s than omega-6s. Another bonus: they contain amino acids like tryptophan and tyrosine, which, as you know, your body needs to make serotonin and dopamine. Beans also contain B vitamins, including folate, and your body needs these to convert amino acids into mood-boosting neurotransmitters.

Another affordable protein source to try as you cut back on meat is whey and casein protein—especially grass-fed or organic varieties. Whey protein helps you to burn calories during the day, and casein protein is great before bed, as it helps you retain lean muscle while you sleep. Pea protein powder is another fantastic choice for both vegans and meat eaters. Mix these protein powders with berries or vegetables along with organic or unsweetened almond milk.

> **RECIPE:** My favorite post-workout shake: vanilla whey protein powder, unsweetened vanilla almond milk, organic blueberries, a handful of kale, a handful of spinach, water, and ice. Try it—it's delicious and filling! See Appendix B, page 247, "A Blender, a Bottle, and a Buck," for more of my favorite smoothies.

And when it comes to spending a few more dollars on organic meat, think of it as a redistribution of your money. Do you save a few dollars at the grocery store and rack up medical bills when all your pro-inflammatory, high omega-6 foods lead to debilitating conditions? Or do you pay a bit more now and save big in the long run by having a healthy and productive life? Remember: you are what you eat.

Also remember that consumer demand causes prices to drop across the board. At the big chain grocery store where I do most of my shopping, there's now enough demand that the chain is marketing its own line of organic eggs, at a much lower price than before. Ditto for the price of organic milk, which seems to go down a bit every time I go to the store. I hope that one day organic becomes the norm and not the exception.

# CHAPTER 6

# A Modified Mediterranean Diet

Chelsea was in her late 20s and worked as a news producer, a job that required her to always be "on" and ready to go at a moment's notice. When she had dinner with a friend or even a date, she kept one eye on her phone to monitor texts, e-mails, and breaking news. Chelsea's body buzzed around the clock with the stress hormone cortisol. Perennially high cortisol levels can lead to low dopamine levels, which was probably why Chelsea felt worn out even after a (rare) good night's sleep.

Chelsea medicated this low-dopamine, low-energy state with caffeine—lots and lots of it. She sometimes drank 10 or 12 cups of coffee, a few diet sodas, and an occasional energy drink to get through a long day. On the days when she actually had time to eat lunch, Chelsea would eat a turkey sandwich and chips from the deli in the lobby.

As they say, "What goes up must come down." At night, alcohol helped Chelsea unwind. After all the coffee and excess stress, she often needed three or sometimes even four glasses of wine to take the edge off. Her dinner was usually a few slices of pizza or chicken and rice. If she couldn't sleep, she'd take some Benadryl. Of course, she'd then wake up groggy and need four cups of coffee before she even got to work, and the cycle would start all over again.

Too much coffee and wine is a problem in and of itself. But the root of Chelsea's problem was her diet, which lacked a variety of vegetables, whole fruits, and healthy proteins that provide the vitamins, cofactors, and amino acids that her brain needed for sustainable energy. Without the folate, vitamin B12, vitamin C, vitamin D, calcium, tryrosine, and omega-3s from spinach, broccoli, blueberries, kale, organic eggs, and wild salmon, Chelsea's body was struggling to make the dopamine she needed to get through her day. With healthier dopamine and energy levels, she wouldn't need so much coffee. Without so much coffee, she wouldn't need so much wine. Without so much caffeine and alcohol, her sleep quality would improve. She'd wake up feeling rested. No wonder she always felt so tired. For Chelsea, too much coffee and wine were merely symptoms of the true problem. In moderation, coffee and red wine are actually two of the most brain-healthy beverages. In excess, they wreak havoc in the brain and body.

After her first session with me, Chelsea made what felt like a very doable change. She bought a few bags of frozen vegetables and fruits and started making some smoothies. A blueberry, kale, spinach, and vanilla protein smoothie was a great lifesaver when she was stuck in the field producing a piece. Just a simple morning drink helped her to go from an average of one to two servings of vegetables and fruits a day to seven. These shakes also served as a great supplement to making time for *real food,* which only happened after I helped Chelsea reframe her priorities.

I told her that missing a news story every once in a while was okay if it meant putting her health first. While Chelsea was in fair health at the time, she simply couldn't keep up her current lifestyle for many more years.

Getting off the upper-downer roller coaster helped Chelsea tremendously. While she had a minor headache for the first few days as her body readjusted to healthy amounts of caffeine, it quickly passed. With more sustainable energy from food, Chelsea no longer needed to rely on excess coffee. And because she was having just two to three cups of coffee or green tea a day, she didn't need the three or four glasses of wine and Benadryl at night to fall asleep. One glass of pinot noir at dinner with a friend felt much better than a bottle of wine watching TV on the couch by herself.

Chelsea benefited greatly from learning that there were long-term solutions to the problems she was facing. Yes, her job was—and always would be—stressful. But by changing the way she lived, she achieved a state of equanimity that would help her weather any storm.

## DIET: THE BIG PICTURE

We have already gone over a number of easy dietary changes that will benefit your brain over the long run: eating complex carbohydrates that don't spike blood sugar, upping your fish intake, and cooking with olive oil. As it happens, many of these habits are pillars of the famous Mediterranean diet, which people in Greece, Italy, and Spain have been adhering to for centuries, with amazing health outcomes. Eating the Mediterranean way can lower the risk of chronic health conditions, cardiovascular disease, and Parkinson's and Alzheimer's as well.

Another Mediterranean secret to living longer and staying slimmer is to eat lots and lots of fruits and vegetables, all day every day. Mediterranean people also avoid getting empty calories from beverages, and instead focus on two of the brain-healthiest beverages out there: coffee and wine.

## FRUITS AND VEGETABLES: LUCKY NUMBER 7

For years, experts have preached that we should all eat five servings of fruits and vegetables every day for optimum health. Then, in 2013, a study looked at over 80,000 people to see how their fruit and vegetable consumption correlated with feelings of happiness. It found that people who eat *seven* servings of fruits and vegetables per day were happier, less nervous, and less frequently depressed.[1]

This makes sense for so many reasons. Fruits and vegetables have potent anti-inflammatory and antioxidant effects that protect the brain.

They support neurogenesis and contain a variety of different vitamins that have been shown to help us think and feel better. This is especially true for vegetables and berries, which deliver brain-protective elements without sending blood sugar sky high like some fruits or fruit juice. (As you'll see on page 166, berries are especially good for protecting cognition in later years, preventing "senior moments," and delaying dementia. Even if you're not to the point where you're worrying about age-related mental health yet, you should definitely read this.)

In terms of feeling better, B vitamins, vitamins A, C, D, and E, calcium, and iodine have all been linked to improved mood, cognition, and energy. As a general principle, the more produce you eat, the more likely you'll be getting the full range of vitamins and minerals that your body and brain need to thrive.

The problem is that the average American is getting just *three* servings of fruits and vegetables a day. (Potatoes, which have a high glycemic index, don't count!) When we don't get enough fruits and vegetables, we end up with vitamin and mineral deficiencies, and when we have these nutritional deficiencies, we don't think or feel our best. The following vitamins are some of the most crucial for brain health and mood stability.

## What to Get: Folate

This B vitamin plays such a big role in feeling better that it's now available as a prescription used to treat depression. But instead of taking a pill, you can get your folate fix with all the vegetables you'll be eating during the 7-Day Energy Revolution. You may be familiar with folic acid, the synthetic form of folate found in fortified products like cereal and other grains. But most Americans are eating way too many carbohydrates, which can lead to brain fog and weight gain. A better solution is to get more folate from something almost everyone could afford to eat more of: vegetables. Research shows that folate can increase the concentration of DHA omega-3s in the bloodstream. It can fight depression, brain fog, dementia, and Alzheimer's by enhancing neurogenesis and decreasing inflammation.[2]

**Where to Get It**: Spinach, Brussels sprouts, romaine, asparagus, and broccoli all contain high levels of folate. So do legumes like lentils, kidney beans, and black-eyed peas.

## What to Get: Vitamin B12

About 40 percent of people between the ages of 26 and 83 have low levels of B12, and 20 percent of patients hospitalized for depression have low levels of the vitamin, which is indispensable for supporting mood, energy, and cognition.[3]

**Where to Get It**: Organic eggs and fish are a fantastic source of vitamin B12.

## What to Get: Vitamin D

If you're inside all day—or eating a lot of conventionally raised meat and not enough fish—you're probably deficient in vitamin D. In fact, new research shows that about 75 percent of American adolescents and adults don't get nearly enough of this think-and-feel-better vitamin.[4] And a recent analysis of 14 different studies found that the lower the subjects' vitamin D levels, the more depressed they felt.[5] Vitamin D is also essential for the proper absorption of calcium, and calcium deficiency itself can lead to anxiety and depression.

**Where to Get It:** Salmon has the most vitamin D of any food, and wild varieties contain far more than polluted, farm-raised varieties. Fruits and vegetables also contain vitamin D, which is why we'll be upping the amount of produce we get in the first week. From now on, seven a day is our new golden rule. Fifteen to twenty minutes of sun exposure is another great way to get vitamin D.

## UNDERSTANDING COFACTORS

A lot of people look at the recommendation to eat seven servings of fruits and vegetables a day and think it's crazy. So instead, they decide to supplement their lower intake with a pill. However, there are many reasons you can't get the benefits of a well-balanced diet in pill form. One is that our bodies need something known as *cofactors* to maximize the nutrition we get out of everything we eat. Cofactors are helper molecules that your body needs to transform amino acids, which you get from the foods you eat, into feel-good neurochemicals like serotonin and dopamine.

Let's look at a very simplified diagram of serotonin and dopamine and how they're made after you eat a meal of plain quinoa, which is definitely one of the best carbs for your health—especially if you pair it with the right foods:

> *Tryptophan (an amino acid found in quinoa)* → *5-HTP (an amino acid and serotonin precursor)* → *serotonin (the anxiety-relieving neurotransmitter)*

But wait! Your body has trouble with this conversion process if it lacks the cofactor "helper molecules." What happens when your body doesn't have enough vitamin B6 from bananas and magnesium from Swiss chard? Your body can't easily convert that tryptophan from the quinoa into the 5-HTP that becomes serotonin.

Of course, the problems don't end there. Low serotonin levels are associated with anxiety and sadness. Serotonin also metabolizes into melatonin, which helps you sleep. So if you're not getting enough serotonin, you might also have trouble getting rested. (This is especially true as you age and melatonin production slows down.) So if you really want to think and feel better, you should combine that quinoa with other fruits and vegetables that support your brain.

*Tryptophan (from quinoa) → vitamin B6 (from bananas) → magnesium (from Swiss chard) → 5-HTP → serotonin (FEEL BETTER) → melatonin (SLEEP BETTER)*

Now let's look at the dopamine you get from having a hard-boiled egg for breakfast:

*Tyrosine (an amino acid found in organic eggs) → L-dopa (an amino acid and dopamine precursor) → dopamine (the depression-relieving neurotransmitter)*

Okay, so where do the cofactors come in? What happens when your body doesn't have enough iron from spinach, vitamin C from yellow bell peppers, and folate from asparagus? Your body has trouble converting the tyrosine in those organic eggs into the L-dopa that turns into dopamine.

Low dopamine is associated with depression, ADHD, and addictive behaviors. The trouble doesn't stop there, either. Dopamine metabolizes into other feel-good neurotransmitters like norepinephrine, but to make that conversion, it needs copper. So what if, instead of plain eggs, you had a delicious omelet with a range of different vegetables?

*Tyrosine (from organic eggs) → iron (from spinach) → vitamin C (from yellow bell peppers) → folate (from asparagus) → L-dopa → dopamine (THINK BETTER, FEEL BETTER) → copper (from mushrooms) → norepinephrine (THINK BETTER, FEEL BETTER)*

And voilà—just like that, you have fed your brain everything it needs for you to function optimally until lunch. Of course, these are just some examples of the cofactors your body and brain depend on. By eating a variety of vegetables and whole fruits every day, you'll be ensuring you're getting the most out of your food.

## GETTING YOUR CAFFEINE FIX

So what about caffeine? In some parts of the Mediterranean (ciao, Italia!), coffee is a huge part of the culture. As Mediterranean people have learned, drinking the right type of caffeine in reasonable quantities can be a great defense against brain fog, and a secret weapon in improving your daily life—and the long-term health of your brain. Caffeine on its own doesn't raise your blood sugar like high-GI carbohydrates do, but it does provide your brain with a jolt of (often much-needed) temporary energy.

Unfortunately, too many people eschew natural sources of caffeine for regular sodas, which, as we've already seen, can spike your blood sugar and fog up your brain. Artificial sweeteners might be even worse, since they can also disrupt the levels of good bacteria in your gut, affecting your mood and cognition.

Energy drinks are perhaps the most dangerous form of artificial caffeine, and we're drinking *way* too many of them. A recent study found that 30 to 50 percent of children and young adults are consuming these drinks, which contain sky-high concentrations of caffeine. (5-Hour Energy contains about 200 mg of caffeine, compared to the 100 mg in a cup of coffee, 60 mg in an espresso, and 40 to 60 mg in green and black teas.) There were over 5,000 caffeine overdose cases in 2007, almost half of those in people younger than 19.[6] Our appetite for caffeine is so voracious that Wrigley developed a gum called Alert Energy Caffeine Gum, which was yanked off the market due to FDA concerns.

But caffeine itself isn't the problem; it's actually quite good for you in the form of unsweetened coffee or tea. As people all over the Mediterranean know, coffee is a health food—the number-one source of antioxidants in the American diet—and can prevent oxidative damage of brain cells and inflammation. Caffeine also protects against cognitive decline and can prevent dementia and Alzheimer's, and drinking coffee actually *decreased* people's risk of depression.[7] If you don't have any health conditions that prevent you from drinking it, you should absolutely drink a little unsweetened coffee or green or black tea every day.

But remember: many of the health benefits of the caffeine in coffee are voided when you mix it with too much blood sugar–spiking sugar, gut bacteria–disrupting artificial sweeteners, or conventional dairy. My two favorite coffee drinks are an espresso macchiato (which contains just a few added calories in the form of foamed milk) and an espresso over ice with a splash of soymilk. Both drinks are under 50 calories and won't spike your blood sugar. (Added bonus: at Starbucks, the soymilk is organic, whereas the regular dairy milk is not.)

But coffee is not a substitute for other important elements in our diets; one reason it's our main source of antioxidants is that most Americans aren't consuming nearly enough spinach, tomatoes, and kale. And too much coffee can be a bad thing. Like a sugar rush, a caffeine high often comes immediately before a resounding crash, leaving us craving either sugar, caffeine, or both to get going again. Like sleep deprivation, caffeinated beverages can interfere with our health, mood, and basic ability to function.

A Mayo Clinic study made headlines for its finding that people under the age of 55 who drink four or more cups of coffee per day faced a 21 percent increased risk of mortality.[8] But another study found that coffee can reduce the risk of dementia and Alzheimer's disease by 65 percent in people who drink between three and five cups per day.[9] Remember: a cup is eight ounces. The average mug or a tall Starbucks cup is 12 ounces. A venti Starbucks is 24 ounces or three cups.

It's a bit confusing since these two ranges overlap a bit, so I recommend that you stick to three cups of coffee a day to enjoy the benefits of caffeine without the risks. In the 7-Day Energy Revolution, we will be scaling down even more, to just two cups a day, for the early weeks of getting our brain back on track.

## RED, RED WINE

We've already seen the surprising brain benefits of drinking a little wine every evening, such as managing blood-sugar spikes. For a non-alcoholic, having up to about one drink per day for women and up to two for men may help keep toxins out of the brain! In one study, scientists gave rats a little bit of alcohol on a daily basis, then introduced a toxin. The result: almost no damage to the brain. But if a rat didn't get this small daily serving of alcohol, damage resulted.

And it's not just in animal studies. A review of 143 studies showed that having up to one drink per day in women and two in men reduced risk of both dementia and Alzheimer's by 23 percent. This benefit held for all types of alcohol, though some studies showed that wine provided more benefits.[10] Another study of over 4,000 people in three different countries showed decreased inflammation in people who reported light to moderate—about one to two drinks per day—alcohol consumption.[11] (By contrast, heavy drinking, defined as more than three to four drinks per day, was associated with an increased risk of dementia and cognitive impairment.)

While these studies showed that the benefits came from the alcohol itself, some of the best benefits come from the skins of grapes. Red wine contains a potent antioxidant called resveratrol, and among red wines, pinot noir has very high levels. The phenolic acid in champagne may also prove a powerful weapon to help you think better. If your dinner drink is a cocktail, stay away from blood sugar–spiking mixed drinks that can wreak havoc on your brain. Trade in gin and tonic for vodka and soda with an extra squeeze of fresh lemon or lime.

> **RECIPE:** For a real treat, try my favorite extra-skinny, frozen strawberry margarita recipe. It uses whole strawberries, which happen to be one of the absolute best fruits for your brain. (See page 166 for the reasons why.) Put 1½ ounces of tequila, 6 ounces soda water, 6 fresh mint leaves, 4 organic strawberries (fresh or frozen), and 1 cup of ice in the blender, then blend and serve. It's delicious!

Drinking one or two servings of alcohol a day can also help decrease inflammation, which in turn can boost your mood, since depression and inflammation are linked. To really maximize the feel-better effects, use some combination therapy by having that glass of wine with a friend to improve your feeling of connection.

However, if you have a personal or family history of alcoholism, problematic alcohol use, or binge drinking, the risks of drinking outweigh the benefits. And not to worry: the other changes you'll be making will produce the same positive results.

## Italy Meets India

While not a Mediterranean staple, turmeric is another essential ingredient to add to your diet. Researchers believe this spice that gives curries their bright yellow color also plays a big role in Indians' low Alzheimer's rates. Curcumin, the active ingredient in turmeric, is a powerful antioxidant and anti-inflammatory that has been linked to improved performance on memory tests.[12] Turmeric might also block the accumulation of the amyloid plaque that's associated with Alzheimer's disease. So, for your brain's sake, make an effort to start eating more turmeric—incorporating small quantities into meals as often as you can.

Just make sure you combine it with pepper—as the Indians do in curry—to make it readily bioavailable, meaning more easily used by the body. One of my favorite ways of getting my turmeric fix is my morning wellness shot. I combine a half teaspoon of turmeric and black pepper with an ounce of cold water and drink it before my coffee. For an extra eye-opening boost, I toss these two ingredients in my blender with fresh lemon juice, cayenne pepper, and ginger.

## YOU ARE WHAT YOU EAT

As we've seen in example after example in this section, diet is everything. Making the right food choices can go a long way toward protecting your brain. By adding more fruits and vegetables to your diet, making an effort to eat more fish, and switching to organic foods whenever possible (especially with animal products), you will be well on your way to thinking and feeling better.

In the next section, we will go beyond food to look at how other aspects of our lifestyles—our sedentary habits, our overreliance on medications, the prevalence of toxins in our environment, and our round-the-clock dependence on technology—also have negative effects on our brains.

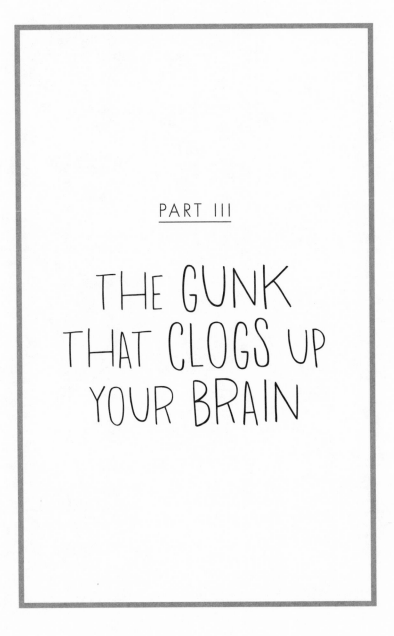

PART III

# THE GUNK THAT CLOGS UP YOUR BRAIN

CHAPTER 7

# Too Many Meds

Jennifer was a personable woman who had just turned 50 and taught history at a small private college. While she felt fulfilled at work, home was a different story. And she had started taking more and more pills to fill a growing emptiness.

The last of her two children had left for college that fall, and Jennifer was suddenly confronting a drastically different life. She'd been married for 25 years, but she felt that the love between her and her husband had been gone for about 15 of those. Early on, she'd confronted her husband about his affairs, but now she just looked the other way. Jennifer knew he had a girlfriend now, but she didn't know what she could do about it.

When I asked why she was still with her husband, she instantly replied, "For the kids, of course. I wouldn't want to upset them."

But Jennifer's problems went much deeper than her husband's infidelity. With her kids gone, she reported that she had very little to look forward to except going to work. She was experiencing a growing malaise and sense of anxiety.

Jennifer had been taking antidepressants, antianxiety meds, and prescription sleeping pills for 15 years—starting around the same time she first caught her husband cheating on her. Her depression had contributed to overeating and high cholesterol. A few years ago, her doctor put her on statins.

Lately, she noticed she needed an extra Xanax to get through the day, and the thoughts spinning in her head at bedtime left her popping Ambien more frequently as well. Over the years, she'd come to have fewer close friends, as her anxiety made her withdraw into the safety of her living room.

This was her very first time going to therapy. Five minutes after meeting her for the first time, I had a strong suspicion that I knew exactly where Jennifer's mild depression and anxiety were coming from. And they weren't problems that prescription medications could remedy.

"Jennifer, what do you need to change in your life to be happy?"

"Well, I guess winning the lottery would be nice. Or maybe if one of the textbooks I wrote became a bestseller that earned me millions of dollars."

"What about something more realistic, but also more scary? Tell me how your life would be different if you were in a loving relationship."

Jennifer began to cry as I asked her to imagine what a loving, supportive relationship might feel like. How much medication would she need then? "None," she replied confidently.

You see, Jennifer wasn't creating a life based on her real desires. She'd built her life around fear.

Yes, divorce is a scary transition. Yes, it's difficult for children initially. But the best gift—both for Jennifer *and also for her children*—is for Jennifer to build a meaningful and happy life. She had plenty of objections. "Who'd want a 50-year-old divorcée?" she asked me. "How would I enter the dating world? Where would I live?"

None of Jennifer's answers would be found in an orange bottle. While some people who experience panic attacks, debilitating insomnia, and major depression do need psychiatric medications, which can be lifesaving, Jennifer was not one of them. For her, medication was numbing her to the joys and possibilities of life. She was choosing short-term avoidance of discomfort over long-term happiness. As a poet once wrote, "The only way around is through." For Jennifer, medicating herself was "going around." I was going to help her "through."

I started by helping Jennifer enrich her personal relationships. This included more time with friends to give her the social support she would need to prevent loneliness during some very big changes in her life. If you focus on adding to people's lives, it becomes easier to take away whatever is holding them back—a key principle in my program.

The lifestyle changes, such as a brain-healthy diet, exercise, and meditation, made Jennifer feel happier and less anxious. She began to reconnect with friends she had neglected, and she started to feel much better about herself. As she became happier, she went back to her primary care doctor and tapered off some of her medications.

Thanks to the changes she made, Jennifer started to feel like maybe her best years were actually *in front of her*. A year later, she filed for divorce. Three years after that, she remarried a wonderful man who would never dream of cheating on her. Jennifer had gotten rid of the blocks that prevented her from feeling clear minded and healthy. In the end, this led to the ultimate reward: love and happiness.

## MORE MEDICATION, MORE PROBLEMS

Many of the medications we routinely take—antidepressants, anti-anxiety meds, sleep aids, stimulants, antipsychotics, and blood-pressure and anti-cholesterol drugs—are essential both for psychiatric problems like depression and for other disorders, like high blood pressure. Yet in my opinion (not to mention the opinion of some of America's most respected experts), we Americans are overmedicated. We are taking medications *far* more frequently and at far higher doses than we really need.

Overmedication can have potentially disastrous effects on our brains. Antidepressants, for example, may increase the risk of inflammation in the brain, and, as we've learned, an inflamed brain ages more rapidly and thinks less clearly. We simply can't think and feel our best when our brains are struggling with inflammation.

## The Polypharmacy Phenomenon

Another disturbing aspect of these medicines is known as the "polypharmacy," in which one medication creates side effects that induces the doctor to prescribe a second medication, which in turn produces side effects that lead to the prescription of a third medication, and so on. This phenomenon reminds me of that song about the old lady who swallowed a fly, then swallowed a spider to catch the fly, then swallowed a bird to catch the spider, and then swallowed a cat to catch the bird . . . all the way on up to swallowing a horse, at which point "she was dead, of course!" While it doesn't usually pose such an immediate risk of death, polypharmacy definitely disrupts our brain chemistry and can put us at risk for dementia and serious brain problems down the line.

There's also a possible association between antidepressants and cancer, and between antianxiety pills and dementia. In fact, all of these increasingly common psychiatric medications can harm the brain, especially when taken regularly over long periods of time by people who don't really need them:

- **Antianxiety meds:** Atarax, Ativan, BuSpar, Catapres, Centrax, Dalmane, Dormalin, Halcion, Inderal, Klonopin, Librium, Neurontin, Paxipam, Prosom, Restoril, Serax, Tenex, Tenormin, Tranxene, Valium, Versed, Vistaril, Xanax

- **Antidepressants:** Adapin, Anafranil, Asendin, Aventil, Celexa, Cymbalta, Desyrel, Edronax, Effexor, Elavil, Lexapro, Ludiomil, Luvox, Marplan, Nardil, Norpramin, Pamelor, Parnate, Paxil, Prozac, Remeron, Serzone, Sinequan, Strattera, Surmontil, Tofranil, Viibryd, Vivactil, Wellbutrin, Zoloft

- **Sleeping Pills:** Ambien, Benadryl, Dalmane, Doral, Edluar, Halcion, Intermezzo, Lunesta, Prosom, Restoril, Rozerem, Silenor, Sonata, Zolpimist

- **Stimulants:** Adderall, Concerta, Cylert, Daytrana, Dexedrine, Focalin, Metadate, Methylin, Nuvigil, Provigil, Ritalin, Sparlon, Vyvanse

- **Antipsychotics:** Abilify, Clozaril, Compazine, Fanapt, Geodon, Haldol, Loxitane, Moban, Navane, Orap, Proketazine, Prolixin, Risperdal, Saphris, Serentil, Seroquel, Solian, Stelazine, Taractan, Thorazine, Tindal, Trilafon, Vesprin, Zyprexa

Every year in the U.S., over 250 million antidepressant prescriptions are dispensed, with about 50 million for Xanax, 27 million for Ativan, and 40 million for Ambien. Add those numbers and they far exceed the population of the country—and this shocking figure doesn't even account for the people who take these medications without a prescription.

## Reading the Labels

Are you finding it hard to believe that these trusted medicines can really be contributing to brain fog, scatterbrain, and memory loss? Well, don't take my word for it—just read the labels. Many warn against "grogginess" or "sleepiness" as possible side effects. Some suggest avoiding driving or operating heavy machinery while under their influence. It's one thing to risk the health of your brain when you are taking a medication that's absolutely critical to your physical, mental, or emotional health. But many of us are taking meds we don't even need!

A whopping two-thirds of Americans currently on antidepressants do not meet the clinical criteria for depression. Yes, these people need help to feel better, but the vast majority of them do *not* need antidepressants, which have serious side effects that could be making their problems worse.

## UNDERSTANDING THE RISKS*

You might be thinking, *But antidepressants—and other drugs on the rise in this country, like Adderall and antipsychotics—are all legal. They're not dangerous like illegal drugs, right?* Wrong. Overdose deaths from prescription painkillers have tripled over the past ten years. These drugs now kill more Americans than heroin and cocaine combined. Emergency room visits for benzodiazepine abuse (e.g., Xanax, Klonopin) surged 89 percent between 2004 and 2008.[1]

Many of these drugs are also addictive, with people gradually increasing their dosage to achieve the same effect. Half a Xanax becomes a full one, then two. Then you go through a stressful breakup and you're popping six. At what point is this medication hurting more than it's helping?

There are problems associated with all four of the most-used psychiatric meds today: antianxiety medications, SSRI and SNRI antidepressants, ADHD stimulants, and Ambien (which we will discuss in detail in Chapter 10, "Light, Sleep, and Technology"). So before you reflexively turn to a prescription pill to cure whatever ails you, first get acquainted with the risks—and the alternatives.

## ANTIANXIETY MEDICATIONS

In 1960, the benzodiazepine Valium hit the U.S. market, followed by other popular benzodiazepines like Klonopin and Ativan. These drugs were an instant sensation among housewives—so popular that the Rolling Stones wrote a song called "Mother's Little Helper" about a woman who uses them simply to get through her day. By 1975, over 100 million benzodiazepine prescriptions were written every year in the U.S.

The troublesome research that began to pop up as early as 1963 didn't seem to make a dent in benzos' popularity. In 1984, scientists

---

* In this section, I will use the name brand to talk about these medications since that is how most people are familiar with these medications. However, I will also use the name brand and generic equivalents interchangeably.

noticed shrunken and damaged brains in the scans of patients who used·benzodiazepines regularly.[2] They also found a link between long-term benzodiazepine use and an increased risk of dementia.[3] Some of the brain-fogging effects of benzodiazepine have been shown to be potentially irreversible, with the subjects in one study continuing to show deficits in verbal learning and memory even after they stopped taking the drug.[4]

Today, scientists are well acquainted with the dangers of benzo-diazepines. In a 2004 meta-analysis, researchers cited several studies of long-term benzodiazepine use affecting several cognitive func-tions, including nonverbal memory impairment, loss of fine motor coordination, and deficits in verbal memory and learning, attention, visuospatial abilities, general intellectual ability, reaction time, psy-chomotor speed, and increased cognitive decline.[5] High doses may result in depression.[6] The authors did find some studies that identified no relationship between long-term benzodiazepine use and cognitive effects, but are *you* willing to take that risk?

Getting off or even reducing the dosage of these drugs has been shown to be extremely difficult as well.[7] As one researcher put it, "It is more difficult to withdraw people from benzodiazepines than it is from heroin."

Given all these risks, concerns about benzos should have become moot when the somewhat less risky SSRIs (selective serotonin reuptake inhibitors) popped onto the American market in 1987. Many of these serotonin-boosting medications effectively treat anxiety without the same risks of abuse, dependence, or dementia.

While many patients did indeed switch to these safer drugs, the maker of the newer benzodiazepine Xanax adopted a clever market-ing strategy to keep benzos relevant: they secured FDA approval to use the drug for panic attacks, and then advertised Xanax as "The First and Only Medication Indicated for Panic Disorder." (Studies had shown that Xanax did indeed help with panic attacks in the first four weeks—but then, when the patients tapered off around week eight, their panic was 350 percent worse, and they also felt more anxious in general compared to the group taking a placebo.)[8]

When the FDA approved Xanax for panic attacks, psychiatrists and psychologists from several countries published a scathing letter condemning the decision. But even with these well-respected medical authorities screaming their disapproval, the marketing worked— big time. Today, more than 50 million prescriptions for Xanax and its generic formulations are filled in this country every year.

Since long-term benzodiazepine use may result in irreversible damage, people with mild to moderate anxiety should first consider cognitive behavioral therapy or other clinically proven models of psychotherapy, changes in diet and exercise, and spiritual practices like meditation—all of which we'll be doing in this program. Drugs this powerful should always be used in combination with therapy, which helps treat the root causes of anxiety and in the process helps reduce or eliminate the amount of medication needed.

## Treating Anxiety

I have treated hundreds of patients with panic attacks, anxiety, PTSD, and phobias. I use graded exposure therapy and other forms of cognitive behavioral therapy to help them make changes that correct the root of the problem, which can "cure" the problem as opposed to just medicating the symptom.

By working in baby steps, I help my patients create real-life experiences that teach them that they can indeed speak in public, get through that meeting without a panic attack, or even reenter the dating world. Medication can sometimes help graded exposure therapy work more effectively; the tapering off starts when they have actually begun to conquer their fears. I, of course, also want them to consider their diet, as high levels of omega-3s may reduce anxiety by 20 percent.

## AN EPIDEMIC OF ANTIDEPRESSANTS

The modern era of antidepressant medication kicked off in 1987 with the introduction of the SSRI Prozac onto the market. Other drug companies quickly brought out competitor SSRIs like Paxil and Zoloft and later Lexapro, Luvox, Celexa, and Viibryd. The 1990s saw the introduction of the serotonin-norepinephrine reuptake inhibitor (SNRI) class, which includes drugs like Effexor, Pristiq, and Cymbalta; these drugs target both serotonin and norepinephrine, another neurotransmitter associated with depression.

According to the CDC, prescriptions for antidepressants tripled from 1988 to 2000. By 2011, there were *264 million* antidepressant prescriptions filled in the U.S. After cholesterol-lowering meds, SSRIs have become the most prescribed class of medication in the country.

On some level, these numbers come as no surprise, since depression is already the leading cause of medical disability in the U.S.[9] It is also—and I can't emphasize this enough—a real disease that requires real treatment. For people who meet the diagnostic criteria for major depressive disorder, antidepressants and clinically proven models of therapy such as cognitive behavioral therapy are as vital as insulin is to a diabetic. Untreated depression can be both debilitating and life threatening.

I will say it again: Depression is a real disease and must be treated as such. If a severely depressed person starts taking antidepressants, he or she should also be in therapy. And in the case of depression, cognitive behavioral therapy has been shown to be extremely effective in achieving remission as quickly as possible.[10] Therapy also helps the patient deal with self-defeating thoughts while providing weekly monitoring for suicidality, which is especially important in kids and teens.

Unfortunately, the nature of depression prevents many who are truly suffering—perhaps even half of all depressed Americans, according to one study—from seeking treatment, which is understandable since depression robs people of energy, motivation, and hope.[11] The depressed brain is also more susceptible to self-loathing, which leads people to characterize their condition as a character defect. Another problem is that depressed people often view asking for help as a sign of weakness, so they stay silent even when they desperately need support.

The flip side of this tragedy is that many of the people who *do* take antidepressants—up to two-thirds of them, in fact—aren't actually depressed. That means that only about 83 million of the 250+ million SSRI prescriptions dispensed every year in this country may be truly necessary.

If you're taking antidepressants and you don't need them, you may be setting yourself up to think and feel worse, with no real benefit. SSRIs come with some well-known side effects, one or more of which most patients will experience: weight gain (ten pounds or more in about 25 percent of patients), sexual dysfunction (which about 50 percent or, in some reports, even more experience), nausea, fatigue, and insomnia.[12]

Constant fatigue is one of the biggest side effects of antidepressants, which can suppress one of your most important functions in terms of rest and memory consolidation: REM sleep. If you're not getting enough REM sleep at night, you're probably feeling tired all day.[13] Also, because they depress REM sleep, prescription antidepressants may interfere with the receptors in your brain getting the rest they need at night, which allows them to regain sensitivity to serotonin and other feel-good chemicals during the day.[14]

Another issue is that while the benefits of SSRIs might take a month to six weeks to kick in, many of the side effects emerge right away. So a person who is already depressed must often "put up" with things getting worse before they get better. And what about when the time comes to change the dose or stop taking the medication? Discontinuing SSRIs can produce irritability, anxiety, and fatigue. And major changes in dosages double the risk of suicide.[15]

Several studies have also identified an alarming association between antidepressants and cancer, especially breast or ovarian cancer.[16] SSRIs can also prevent anticancer drugs from working well in patients, which has been shown to lead to an increased risk of death in women being treated for cancer while also taking an antidepressant.[17]

There is also an increased risk of death and stroke. A 2009 study looked at over 100,000 postmenopausal women—a group that is fairly likely to be taking antidepressants—over at least five years and found that the women taking antidepressants were much more likely to have a stroke or die compared to women not taking antidepressants. Both newer SSRIs and the older tricyclic antidepressants showed this risk.[18]

But surely these hazards are all par for the course, right? These drugs must be remarkably effective if they're prescribed so frequently; otherwise, doctors wouldn't bother. Maybe—or maybe not. In 2007, the esteemed *New England Journal of Medicine* looked at both published and unpublished studies on the effectiveness of antidepressants. All but one of the studies with a favorable outcome had been published, whereas *half* of the studies that failed to show a favorable outcome never saw the light of day. There was also a nearly one-to-one ratio of total studies, both published and unpublished, that found these drugs to be effective versus those that did not, meaning that for every study that found these drugs worked, another found that they didn't.[19] So really the jury is still out on just how effective these drugs really are—especially for those with less severe forms of depression.

Even where the antidepressants were found to be effective, the placebo effect played a big role—meaning people with minor depressive symptoms responding to antidepressants reported similar improvement by taking a sugar pill. Even those studies that did show antidepressants were effective found that placebos were *82 percent as effective as the drug itself.*[20]

And as evidenced by the huge popularity of these drugs, many people assume that no "natural" treatment could possibly be as effective in treating major depression. Yet one study that compared Prozac to an omega-3 supplement with high levels of EPA found that they were equally effective at controlling depressive symptoms in patients diagnosed with major depression.[21] The difference is that the former is associated with side effects, whereas the latter comes with added health benefits. The other game-changing, drug-free option in treating major depression and other mental illnesses is transcranial magnetic stimulation (TMS) which uses magnetic pulses in 15- to 30-minute sessions to activate the brain. Repetitive transcranial magnetic stimulation (rTMS) and deep transcranial magnetic stimulation (deep TMS) have both received FDA approval for treating major depression in cases where prescription antidepressants have failed.

Research is under way to see if TMS is an effective drug-free treatment for other conditions such as ADHD, bipolar disorder, insomnia, anxiety, addiction, and pain.

## Inflammation and Depression

Antidepressants can also potentially leave you thinking badly and feeling worse by increasing inflammation, which researchers have recently discovered might play a significant role in triggering depression. (While some research has shown antidepressants decrease certain markers of inflammation, other recent studies have indicated antidepressants may actually increase inflammation.)[22] There is some chicken-or-the-egg at play here; inflammation may cause depression or depression may cause inflammation. Either way, the conditions are clearly linked and should be addressed in tandem. You simply cannot treat depression without also taking inflammation into account.

So if you're eating the typical American inflammatory diet of high omega-6s from nonorganic beef or chicken, soybean oil used in most dressings, soda, added sugar, or flour, you might be putting yourself at a greater risk of depression.[23] A massive study of 73,000 people over a span of years found that people with higher markers of inflammation in their blood increased their risk of depression two- to threefold.[24]

Inflammation in the brain can lead to fatigue. The inflammation-depression relationship may also explain why so many nonpsychiatric illnesses are associated with depression. It's not just situational (i.e., feeling sad that you have been diagnosed with an illness) but also biological. The long-term inflammation associated with a nonpsychiatric illness like cancer or autoimmune diseases may put that person at risk for depression as a result of the biologically based inflammation occurring in the body and brain.[25]

With all this troubling new research about antidepressants, we should probably conduct a risk-benefit analysis and reconsider our overreliance on them. I believe that if you suffer from milder forms of depression and anxiety, you owe it to yourself to try a treatment with benefits that can last a lifetime.

## ATTENTION DEFICIT DISORDER DRUGS

Like depression, attention-deficit hyperactivity disorder is a real disease with symptoms that usually surface in childhood and persist into adulthood in about 65 percent of people diagnosed.[26] Also like depression, ADHD requires treatment, and that treatment can often include medication.

For people who truly have ADHD, brain scans show that the long-term use of Adderall—the flagship stimulant used to treat ADHD—can correct the parts involved in attention and inhibition.[27] And helping the child's brain learn will surely have lasting implications for that child's future.

But how many people who take Adderall really have ADHD? And how many of them are simply taking it as a performance enhancer to keep up with their peers or colleagues?

Since the FDA approved Adderall in the 1990s, the numbers of people taking the drug have gone up, up, and away. Tens of millions of Adderall prescriptions are filled every year. With almost $8 billion spent on ADHD meds in 2011 (double the $4 billion just four years before), stimulants are big money. The number of young adults on stimulants also doubled between 2007 and 2011.[28]

And it's not just young people. Adderall has become the "Mother's Little Helper" for a new generation of moms. Gone is the bored *Mad Men*–era housewife who fills her day with martinis and Valium to medicate her loneliness and boredom. The new archetype is the single mom, the working mom, the two-earner-household-but-we-still-can't-make-ends-meet mom. If a little pill helps her get everything done for her family, what could possibly be wrong with it? A lot.

Research shows that Adderall is addictive, with multiple withdrawal effects, and it can be as hard to recover from as heroin addiction.[29] Adderall carries a black box warning and is a schedule-II medication. This puts it in the same category as cocaine, methadone, and morphine. It is an extremely serious medication.

And you don't have to steal it from little Johnny or even find a drug dealer to get your fix. These days, any adult—or even any college student—with Internet access can figure out which symptoms to report to doctors to score a prescription.[30] The new diagnosis manual for psychiatric conditions has eased the diagnostic requirements for adult ADHD, which means Adderall will probably be prescribed even more in years to come.

These days, college campuses all over the country are swimming in Adderall. At some colleges, up to 25 percent of the students use prescription stimulants without a prescription.[31] With so many taking the drug illegally or with a feigned prescription, are students who *don't* take Adderall at a disadvantage? In competitive, ranked fields of study like law and medicine, they might be, and that in itself is a problem.

## ANTIPSYCHOTICS

Antipsychotics are a great example of how direct-to-consumer pharmaceutical commercials—a practice illegal everywhere in the world except the U.S. and New Zealand—have turned unprofitable, rarely used drugs into blockbusters.

With the help of canny ad campaigns, sales of antipsychotic drugs have doubled in the past decade. In children, atypical antipsychotics (newer medications distinguished from the older antipsychotics with expired patents) have risen from 2.9 million prescriptions in 2002 to 4.8 million in 2009. These newer antipsychotics are much more profitable to pharmaceutical companies, as they can sell the name-brand-only formulations. They are, in fact, the most profitable class of psychiatric meds.[32]

But let's never forget that these are serious drugs with serious side effects. Atypical antipsychotics are associated with diabetes, weight gain, and cardiovascular disease. In children, they are increasingly being used off-label to treat ADHD, despite evidence that the children taking these medications are three times more likely to develop type 2 diabetes. Adult diabetics are much more likely to develop dementia.

The cheerful commercials for the very popular Abilify portray the drug as a "mood booster" that will increase happiness. But in reality, this antipsychotic med can do all sorts of damage to the body, including the brain.

The commercials communicate the message that if you are sad or struggling in any way, shape, or form, you should probably be on a psychiatric medication. And it's true that some people really do need medication—but do you? Perhaps the sadness you're experiencing is information that you're in the wrong relationship or the wrong job. Maybe it's an opportunity to make changes in your life that will actually change your mood for good. Maybe you're achy because your muscles are sore, and maybe your back is stiff because you're not moving your body the way it was designed to move. You don't need Abilify; you need a gym membership!

## STATINS AND OTHER NONPSYCHIATRIC MEDICATION

Since cholesterol-lowering statins obtained FDA approval in 1987, they have quickly become one of the most widely used (and most profitable) classes of medications, with a whopping one in four Americans over the age of 55 already on one. And that number is set to increase exponentially in the years to come.

While a heart attack–prevention medicine might appear totally unrelated to thinking and feeling better, statins have been linked to cognitive decline, memory loss, dementia, and Alzheimer's disease. They've also been shown to increase blood sugar, which, as we know, can lead to brain fog and eventually dementia. In postmenopausal women who take statins, there is a 48 percent increased risk of diabetes.[33]

Part of the risk of taking statins—and countless other prescription medications—is that many drugs interfere with the absorption of the nutrients your brain needs to function. Statins deplete the enzyme CoQ10, which is a powerful antioxidant that's necessary for cell growth. Many over-the-counter and prescription medications—including aspirin, antibiotics, antacids, birth control pills and patches, asthma medications, ibuprofen, and steroids—can deplete B vitamins, which are essential for boosting mood and energy.[34]

Even drugs that are considered extremely safe have been linked to conditions that affect the brain. A recent study found a troubling connection between acetaminophen (Tylenol) use in pregnancy and ADHD.[35] And innumerable nonpsychiatric meds have been linked to depression, including beta blockers, anti-Parkinson's drugs, proton-pump inhibitors, hydralazine, efavirenz, antineoplastic agents, hormone-altering drugs, anticonvulsants, H2 blockers, and anticholinergic drugs.[36]

Again, you should *always* take any medication if you genuinely need it. If a statin is going to prevent you from having a heart attack that could end your life, you should obviously continue to take it. But before upping your dosage once again, you might stop to ask yourself if you've already done everything within your power to get your cardiovascular health under control. If the answer is yes and you still need a statin or blood-pressure lowering drug, be sure that you're getting enough of the right nutrients from food to counteract whatever negative effects may be taking place.

Instead, far too many people who take these and other medications feel that their prescription licenses them to eat or do whatever they want, when in fact the opposite is true. People think, *Now that I'm on Prozac, I no longer have to deal with that relationship that made me so sad to begin with.* Or *Now that I'm on this statin, I can have a bacon cheeseburger and a milkshake for lunch every day.* The truth is that when you're on a prescription medication, you should try even harder to maintain a healthy lifestyle.

Even vitamins can be a problem when people take them to compensate for an unhealthy behavior like smoking. This phenomenon may offer a possible explanation to the recent report that people who didn't take vitamins lived slightly longer than those who did: the vitamin takers in the research may have been making more unhealthy choices than those who didn't take vitamins but lived generally healthier. Vitamins and fish oil can work wonders for your health. The trick: use an "and" approach instead of an "or" approach. Take vitamins, psychiatric meds, or statins if needed *and* eat healthy and make good choices as opposed to taking vitamins, psychiatric meds, or statins *or* eating healthy and making good choices.

## TAKING ACTION

There's no quick, one-size-fits-all solution to the problems that have so many of us turning to prescription medications on a far too regular basis, but we can make some lifestyle adjustments to steer us toward a better night's sleep and away from depression, anxiety, and panic. Every recommendation in this book is geared toward long-term solutions that can leave us thinking and feeling better with minimal pharmaceutical interventions.

Anxiety, sadness, or addiction can be telling you that what you're doing in your life isn't working. It may be what you're eating (or not eating), who you're loving (or not loving), or how you're dealing (or not dealing) with life's problems. When you start listening to your emotions and taking the messages they're communicating more seriously, you will start to manifest everyday miracles in your life.

You should also make an effort to reframe moderate amounts of so-called negative emotions like anxiety to realize how they can be helpful. Research shows that moderate anxiety can actually improve performance on tests, increasing concentration and forging new connections in the brain. These bouts of concentration can help prevent cognitive decline and dementia, and they can also increase your happiness by rewarding you with challenging work.

Depression may also be a signal that it's time to change your perception of the world. If, for example, you see everything through the lens of "I'm not okay," you're likely to interpret every ache in your body to mean you have stage 4 cancer. If you view the world through a lens of "I'm not good enough," you incorrectly assume *you* are to blame for every one of life's disappointments.

It's time to examine your life to find evidence that you *are* okay and more than good enough. Start looking for what's right in your life, not what's wrong. Maybe it's not *what* you see in your life but *how* you see it. You'll learn more of these strategies as you embark on my 21-day program.

Even the flashbacks, nightmares, panic attacks, and anxiety that result from trauma are useful information. They're telling you that it's time to seek treatment. Many people medicate their traumas with benzodiazepines or alcohol or both, but trauma—as it relates to a soldier's PTSD or a survivor of sexual abuse—needs reprocessing through psychotherapy. Until people are successfully treated through cognitive behavioral interventions, as opposed to just having their symptoms medicated, lasting relief is unlikely. While antianxiety medication can make the early stages of treatment more successful, the goal is not to stay on medication but rather to work toward extinguishing or minimizing the symptoms *without* medication, or with the smallest dose necessary.

Underneath this American phenomenon of overmedication is a belief that we should never be uncomfortable in any way. On a much deeper level, this conviction comes from fear. Living life and making choices based on fear is no way to invite abundance, joy, and love. For human beings, it is our *experiences* that have the profound power to change the way we think and feel. Is there something scary that you know you need to do in your life to grow? In most cases, that will be far more effective and profound than the persistent medication of symptoms. If you need these medications, let them serve as tools to help you change, not crutches for long-term dependency.

## A LITTLE ORANGE BOTTLE WITH BIG PROBLEMS

I do understand that there's a great deal of psychological power in that little orange bottle. It says, "I'm a heavy hitter. I'll make you feel better. A doctor prescribed me, so I must be good for you." You assume that this pill must obviously be more effective than changes in what you eat or how much light you're exposed to. And if so-called natural remedies worked so well, why don't the big pharmaceutical companies make prescription drugs out of them?

The answer is that in other countries, that's exactly what they do. In Germany, St. John's wort, a natural herb with antidepressant effects, is prescribed far more than Prozac or Paxil. The way U.S. law is set up means you will find herbs and other natural remedies like St. John's wort or turmeric in the food aisle instead of behind the pharmacy counter. And some natural remedies may be more effective in promoting good mood with fewer side effects compared to the drugs in the little orange bottles. In fact, most of the "side effects" of natural solutions like omega-3s include better skin, longer life, and decreased risk of many major diseases.

Speaking of drug-free remedies, what about psychotherapy? From a financial point of view, psychotherapy is far more expensive in the short term than paying for your generic Xanax or Prozac. And while the effects of six months of cognitive behavioral therapy can last a lifetime while the antidepressant effects of Prozac stop when you start taking them, this long-term savings isn't very persuasive to your insurance company. But it's not just your insurer; it's you, too! Complying with therapy or lifestyle changes requires more hard work, commitment, and motivation than popping a pill—but it is well worth the effort.

CHAPTER 8

# Taking On Toxins

Making smart choices about your diet, getting enough sleep, controlling your medications—all of these factors play a crucial role in how your brain functions. But to think and feel your absolute best, you must also take on the toxins in your food, air, and water. By doing so, you'll be addressing the root causes of any problems of low mood or brain fog. It's also part of a whole-person approach to thinking and feeling better.

Many of us don't realize it, but the pesticides and pollutants all around us are fogging and clogging our brains, leading to a whole host of scary symptoms: Lowered IQ. Depression. Anxiety. Hyperactivity. Aggressive behavior. ADHD. Developmental disruption. Diminished intellectual function. Cognitive decline. Dementia. Cancer.

Every year, it seems as if there are more and more environmental toxins out there that can negatively affect the brain. And I'm not just talking the chemicals under your sink with the skull and crossbones on the label. Some are in your fridge and possibly even in your tap water.[1]

Because the government won't protect you from most of these threats, you have the responsibility to reduce your (and your children's) exposure to these pervasive environmental toxins yourself.

## TOXIC DRINKING WATER

Drinking water is essential for maintaining good health, but some water pollutants could be making you think and feel worse.

There are many possible perpetrators: manganese in drinking water, for example, has been linked to hyperactivity and lower math scores in children. While some communities filter manganese out, many don't. To be on the safe side, invest in an inexpensive activated carbon filter water pitcher, which can remove 60 to 100 percent of manganese from your water.[2]

One company, Clear2O, uses an even more effective technology that has been shown to reduce more toxins, including the traces of medications that lurk in a lot of tap water. These filters are also a good defense against the lead—one of the most brain-damaging toxins there is—in some old household water pipes.

Where you store your water might also be an issue. When buying plastic water bottles, look for BPA-free versions. Glass or stainless steel water bottles are an even safer bet, given recent evidence that even BPA-free plastics can contain dangerous toxins.

If you do buy water in disposable plastic bottles, don't let them sit out in your car or garage, since heat makes the chemicals leach from the plastic. This is especially important for children's developing brains, as they're far more vulnerable to damage from toxins.

## YOUR COOKING EQUIPMENT CAN MAKE YOU SICK

Cooking at home is important if you want to control blood-sugar spikes and take charge of your diet, but you should pay attention to what you use to cook. Nonstick cookware is often manufactured with perfluorooctane sulfonate (PFOS) and perfluorooctanoate (PFOA), which have been linked to lower birth weight and smaller head circumference when children are exposed to them in utero.[3] PFOA has also been shown to cause tumors in rats.[4]

While there are some safe, effective ceramic-based nonstick options out there, I would recommend ditching your nonstick cookware in favor of cast iron or stainless steel. If you're still stuck, so to speak, on Teflon, consider some common-sense guidelines. Chemicals begin to break down above 500 degrees, and toxic gases and carcinogens can be released around 680 degrees. So stick to low or medium heat and use heavier pans, which take longer to heat up. Open windows or turn on your hood vent. If the pan's coating is chipped or flaking, throw it out. The older these pans get, the more likely they are to release toxins.

Microwave popcorn bags can also contain the same chemicals as nonstick pans (and the microwave popcorn itself often uses unhealthy oils), so instead use plain kernels and microwave in a brown lunch bag or use an air popper. After popping, drizzle with a tablespoon of extra virgin olive oil and a dash of sea salt.

## STAGNANT INDOOR AIR

The air in our homes might be swirling with any number of invisible toxins—dust mites and bacteria; particles from cooking, cleaning, smoking, and pet dander; pollutants brought in from outdoors like pollen, pesticides, and heavy metals—that can reduce our ability to perform mental tasks and even contribute to diseases as serious as cancer.

To counteract these effects, dust and mop more regularly and use a HEPA filter on your vacuum and heating or cooling systems. You should also wash your hands more frequently to reduce your exposure to these toxins. And make a few little household tweaks as well.

In 2001, the EPA restricted how much lead could be used in paint used in child-care facilities after lead poisoning cases. Still, many paints contain dangerous chemicals that affect the air quality of your house, so consider using environmentally friendly paints when painting your home.

Most important of all, try bringing some nature indoors. Keep your windows open as much as possible, since indoor air is often far dirtier than air outside. Also make an effort to minimize the dirt you bring into your house. Research shows that people who take off their shoes at the front door significantly reduce the amount of dust containing PCB toxins in their home.

Consider putting a few houseplants in every room, since they purify the air while soothing your spirit. Certain plants are better than others at removing toxins like benzene and formaldehyde from the air: areca palm, lady palm, bamboo palm, English ivy, dwarf date palm, Boston fern, and peace lily are especially effective at cleaning the air you breathe.

## CLEANING PRODUCT PROBLEMS

Don't muddy up your brain while cleaning your house. Look for nontoxic cleaning supply options, and choose an environmentally friendly dry cleaner. The dry-cleaning chemical tetrachloroethylene has been linked to a higher risk of psychiatric disorders in children. At the very least, consider taking your clothes out of the plastic wrapping and airing them out outside or in your garage before bringing them into your closet.

You should also be aware of the PBDEs (polybrominated diphenyl ethers) used as a flame retardant in mattresses, carpets, and furniture. PBDEs—classified by the EPA as persistent organic pollutants, as they linger in the body—disrupt your thyroid regulation, which can lead to depression and weight gain. In children, they have been linked to autism, lower IQs, and slower cognitive development.

Lawn care is another area that could be affecting your brain. Carbamates that are sprayed on lawns and used to kill cockroaches have been linked to deficits in children's brain development, so consider your lawn-care options carefully, and think twice before you use harmful chemicals to kill bugs in your home.

There are some simple ways you can minimize the impact of PBDEs. The high-folate and B-vitamin foods you will eat in week 1, the exercise in week 2, and the stress-relieving approaches you'll embrace in week 3 reduce the chances that the PBDEs you encounter will result in health problems for you or developmental defects in your children.

With many toxins, risk factors often combine. For example, a person exposed to PBDEs who eats the food in this program will be less likely to have thyroid disruption than a person exposed to the same amount of PBDEs who lives off junk food. By reducing the toxins in one part of your life, you'll be reducing the risk factors for all of them. Every bit counts.

## THE BIG PICTURE

Much of the advice I prescribe in the rest of the book—eating organic, exercising regularly—specifically applies to warding off these other toxic influences in the environment. That's because the healthier you are in general, the less susceptible you will be to toxins. Managing blood-sugar spikes and increasing exercise will not only reduce brain fog and prevent dementia, but will also help you lose weight, and losing weight helps protect you against toxins because PBDEs and other persistent organic pollutants *accumulate in fat.*

The more excess fat you're carrying, the more toxins you're likely carrying around as well. Toxins accumulate in animal fat, which also means that fattier cuts of meat in nonorganic animal products are more harmful than the leaner ones. When eating nonorganic animal products, favor chicken breast, egg whites, and skim milk over beef, whole eggs, and 2-percent or full-fat milk. These measures will also help you to reduce your intake of omega-6s, which are more concentrated in fattier cuts of nonorganic animal products.

Reducing the amount of fat in your body is a remarkably effective way to reduce the risks related to toxins. So get out there and start exercising—and sweat as much as you can! Your skin is often the first point of contact for many toxins and pollutants. So sweat it out at the gym during your workout. And afterward, fuel up with wild salmon or some of the other high omega-3, low toxin seafood listed on pages 46 to 47. One study showed that fish oil actually protected against some of the adverse effects of being exposed to polluted air.[5]

Living in a bubble may not be an option (nor should it be!), but you can take a lot of simple steps to make your life as clean and healthy as possible. Your body and brain will thank you!

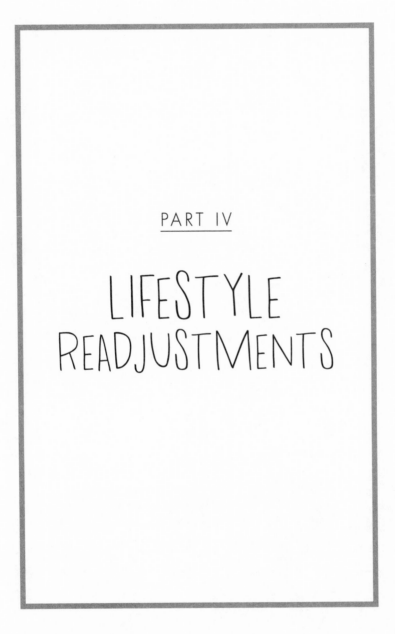

PART IV

# LIFESTYLE READJUSTMENTS

# CHAPTER 9

# Our Way Too Sedentary Lives

Doug was a father of three who lived in a nice four-bedroom house an hour away from his office where he worked as an accountant. He and his wife had moved farther away from the city after their third child was born. Doug definitely enjoyed some aspects of his suburban existence: a bigger house, better public schools, and fewer loud ambulances zooming by in the middle of the night. While Doug was confident that he'd made the right decision for his family, his move to the suburbs wasn't all hunky-dory for him.

Two hours in the car on weekdays added to his long days at work and duties as a dad meant he wasn't getting enough sleep. Romance in his marriage felt like a distant memory; he couldn't even remember the last time he'd had dinner alone with his wife. Doug's energy levels were down, and his weight was up: he had gained 30 pounds in just two years. He tried a no-carb diet for all of ten horrible days. While he did shed a few pounds, he also felt incredibly irritable and hungry. He paid several hundred dollars for a month of unlimited intense group weight-lifting classes, but he made it to only two classes in those 30 days. He also had tried leaving an hour earlier for work to beat the traffic, but his modified schedule made it difficult to interact with colleagues and clients during normal business hours.

Doug was starting to feel as if all the joy had been sucked out of his life. While he loved his wife and kids, he felt too tired to enjoy them or give them the attention they deserved.

"I just don't know what I can do," he told me. "Even if we wanted to, we can't move. The mortgage on our house is more than it's worth. I can't quit my job. Honestly, I just feel so stuck. I can't live like this for the next twenty-five years. Something has to change," Doug said in a hopeless voice.

I gave him an encouraging smile and said, "The good news, Doug, is that I believe the solution is much easier than you think."

Doug's all-or-nothing pattern of problem solving had landed him in trouble. It was my job to help him see the gray-area antidote to his problems. He didn't have to wake up at 4 A.M. or go to a boot camp class every single day to think and feel better. Doug just needed to take a walk at lunch every day and reduce—but not eliminate—the processed carbs in his diet.

As they say, slow and steady wins the race. Doug started to see how simple, sustainable strategies were the secret to success. He started taking the stairs every day at work. A wireless headset for his office phone allowed him to get up and move at least twice an hour. He and his wife planned a weekly date night; feeling more connected to her helped him feel hopeful about his life, which had the unexpected result of boosting his energy. And they walked the half mile to the restaurant instead of driving, which wasn't just exercise; it was a nice chance to spend quality time together and decompress from their day. Doug swapped his afternoon latte and chips for two shots of espresso over ice and a protein bar. Losing a few pounds gave him more energy to play with his kids.

## EXERCISE AND THE BRAIN

How exactly did we become so inactive? Let me count the ways. We travel too far to work, with Americans commuting on average 25 minutes to their jobs every day.[1] More and more of us sit all day once we get there: from 1970 to 2000, the number of Americans in sedentary desk jobs has doubled.[2] And most shocking of all, we watch *way* too much TV. In the early 2000s, Americans spent an average of almost four hours a day watching television.[3] By 2012, that had rocketed up to *five hours and 15 minutes* a day watching TV—a figure that includes live TV, DVR, and DVD, which suggests that we don't replace old technology (live television) with new technology (DVR playback) but just keep on adding to it.[4]

Five-plus hours is already a substantial chunk of time to spend slumped on a couch, but what happens when we add up all the time we devote to browsing the Internet on our iPhones, watching YouTube on our tablets, or online shoe shopping on our laptops? And what about when we engage with two or more media sources simultaneously? That's when it gets really scary. A 2013 report found that the average American spends a whopping *12 hours, five minutes per day with major media,* which includes TV, Internet, phone, radio, and magazines or newspapers.

So what's wrong with watching TV all evening after work, or staying plugged into our smartphones and tablets 24/7? A great deal, actually. One study found that for every two hours spent watching TV, the risk of dying from any cause increased 13 percent, and the risk of developing type 2 diabetes rose 20 percent. The subjects in the study who watched the most television were 61 percent more likely to die compared to those who watched one hour per day.[5]

With every passing year, more and more Americans are considered "inactive" as categorized by the CDC: 36 percent in 2008 and 43.3 percent in 2012.[6] And a 2014 study showed that just 6.2 percent of over 2,000 adults aged 60 and over met the government's standards for physical activity. And every hour they spent sitting increased their risk of being disabled by 50 percent![7]

That's right: by 50 percent. Eye-opening stats like that are one reason sitting has become widely known as the "new smoking" for the harm it does to the body. Scientists have coined the term "sitting disease" to describe the various ill effects associated with sitting for too long: obesity, cardiovascular disease, a nearly 50 percent increased risk of death from any cause. Too much sitting has been linked to a huge range of medical problems, from the skeletal—strained neck, sore shoulders and back, and damaged disks—to the internal: poor circulation, colon cancer, and an overproductive pancreas.[8]

The good news is that you can dramatically improve these outcomes with some extremely simple measures, like taking some light-intensity breaks—the equivalent of just six minutes of walking per hour—during long bouts of sitting. These breaks are especially important immediately after you've eaten, according to one study. After ingesting 760 calories—roughly the amount most of us consume at lunch or dinner—subjects had their blood sugar monitored hourly. On another day, they had the same amount of calories and just did some light walking for six minutes each hour. The result? The blood sugar spiked 20 percent less when people took light breaks.[9] So there's a good physiological reason that so many people enjoy an after-dinner stroll: the body benefits from a little movement after consuming all those calories.

And even if you exercise at high intensity most days (go, you!), you also need to incorporate regular activity into different segments of your day. One 2010 study found that men—even those who routinely exercised—who sat for 23+ hours per week had a 64 percent greater risk of dying from heart disease than those who sat for less than 11 hours.[10] So it's important to move for a few minutes every hour, rather than (or in addition to) in one intense burst.

The more time we spend zoned out in front of the TV, phone, or laptop, the more likely we'll be fogging our brains and bodies. Some of the damage could be offset if we were eating fewer calories, getting more omega-3s and fewer omega-6s, and not constantly spiking our blood sugar. Instead we are taking the opposite course: overdosing on sugars, bread, and nonstop omega-6s. The only answer is to clean up our lifestyles and get moving.

## WHY EXERCISE?

Most of us already know that regular exercise helps to maintain a healthy body weight. But it's probably even more beneficial to our brains than we might've realized. It turns out exercise may be *the single best mood booster out there.* It's extraordinarily effective at boosting energy and combating both anxiety and depression.

In fact, numerous studies have shown that exercise, when done consistently, actually *outperforms* antidepressants in improving mood and cognitive function. It even boosts levels of brain-derived neuro-trophic factor (BDNF), which supports cell growth in the brain, in addition to endorphins and other feel-good chemicals.

One Duke study divided depressed patients into three groups. The first took the popular antidepressant Zoloft; the second exercised for 45 minutes with no Zoloft; the third took Zoloft *and* exercised. Four months later, all three groups had similar positive improvements. Fast forward ten months and what happened? Only 8 percent of the exercisers saw depressive symptoms return, compared with 38 percent of those taking Zoloft and 31 percent of those taking Zoloft *and* exercising.[11]

The catch was that the subjects had to keep up the exercise or the benefits diminished. But the movements involved weren't some intense boot camp exercises. It was simply jogging or stationary bike riding. The message here is that consistency trumps intensity. A 2005 Harvard study found that even walking fast for 35 minutes had a significant impact on depression.

And it's not just *feeling* better but *thinking* better, too. Stimulating BDNF, which promotes neurogenesis while destroying Alzheimer's disease–causing plaques, through exercise is like stem-cell therapy for your brain. It helps create new pathways as you engage in new and challenging experiences.

Again, you don't have to move much to reap big benefits. One study showed that walking just *one mile per day*—that's only about 2,000 steps!—cuts the risk of future memory problems, including cognitive impairment and dementia, by 50 percent.[12] Brain scans showed the mile-a-day walkers had increased volume in the all-so-important brain areas like the hippocampus (central to learning) and the prefrontal cortex (the most advanced part of the brain). In another study of more than 2,000 men, those who walked less than a quarter mile a day were 1.8 times more likely to develop dementia than those who walked the most.[13]

If the benefits of moving are this huge (and the risks of staying still are as well), why not try to incorporate some more basic movements into your days? It is so incredibly easy. You will look better, feel better, and think better, faster than you can walk around the block.

## Leaky Brain: The New Leaky Gut

Our bodies are designed to take in what we need while keeping the bad stuff out. In the case of leaky gut, undigested food and bacteria begin to go where they shouldn't through the lining of your intestines, which triggers symptoms like bloating, inflammation, and fatigue. For people with celiac disease or a gluten sensitivity, this is caused by a molecule called zonulin. A surge of this molecule can make both the gut and the blood-brain barrier—your brain's defense system that keeps the bad stuff out—more permeable to toxins. For years, we've known that gluten sensitivity may make the brain more susceptible to toxins.

But groundbreaking research shows that leaky brain isn't just something that affects people who are sensitive to gluten. People who are obese or sedentary may also be prone to leaky brain—and also more vulnerable to brain fog and depression as a result. A 2014 study found elevated levels of a pro-inflammatory molecule in the blood of obese mice. Even more troubling: this molecule also made its way past the blood-brain barrier and migrated to the brain. Once there, it affected areas associated with learning as well as the synapses associated with healthy mood.[14]

The good news is that when the overweight rats exercised, the inflammation decreased, synaptic health increased, and cognition improved.

## PRESCRIPTION: GET MOVING

Before Facebook and Twitter there was another great American invention: the Ford Model T. It was produced from 1908 to 1927, it was the first automobile that was affordable to the average American. Cars paved the way for suburbs. After World War II, the urban exodus began, and by 1950 more Americans lived in suburbs than in cities.[15]

And with this exodus, commuting—by car and also by train—sky-rocketed. Over the years, commute times have gotten longer as traffic has worsened and home prices in metropolitan areas have increased, forcing more and more people to move even farther away from the city. And, as one study found, driving just ten miles or more to work was associated with high blood sugar, low levels of physical activity, and a higher risk of depression and anxiety.[16]

So it seems that real-estate agents may be right. It truly is all about location, location, location. When I moved last year, I knew *exactly* where I wanted to live. My goal was to find a place within a five-minute walk to my office. I succeeded, and I can now make the one-and-a-half-block walk from my front door to my office in about 100 seconds.

What did I sacrifice for this ultimate convenience? Space, lots of it. In my new home, I have only one bathroom. I don't have central air and heat. But my office is right around the corner, and I'm just three blocks from a great park where I take my dog every day. My favorite grocery store is just two blocks away, too, so I don't even have to get in the car when I run out of milk. The result: I am happier and more peaceful, and I feel connected to the people in my community. I frequently go for days without getting in my car.

My own experience has taught me that living in a walkable neighborhood as close to work as possible is one of the best things you can do to think and feel better, although relocating from your current residence is obviously not an option for most people. But if you're planning to move anyway, consider a home that lends itself to a real walking lifestyle. (There's a website, walkscore.com, that lets you enter any address in the country and it gives you the location's walk score on a scale of 1 to 100, based on the place's proximity to restaurants, services, and public transportation options.)

If a change of address isn't on the horizon for you, you can still make some significant tweaks to your routine. Are there restaurants within walking distance of your house? Try them. Instead of ordering Chinese food delivery, get takeout and pick it up yourself, even if it adds half an hour to your evening—I promise it'll be pleasurable, and you'll probably sleep better afterward. What about that gym that's not quite as big or fancy as the one you belong to now but just a quick ten-minute jog away? Consider switching your membership from the one that's a half hour in the car from your house if it means you'll get there more often.

When you set up your life to make walking a daily priority, you might be amazed by how quickly the changes take place in your body and brain.

## ACTION PLAN

I really can't emphasize it enough: incorporating *a moving lifestyle* is vital to your health. That's why in the 7-Day Energy Revolution, you will commit to just 44 minutes of exercise a day, in one or two sessions. So if you're a busy working mom who hasn't had time to exercise in the three years since you gave birth, you'll take a brisk 22-minute walk at lunch and then jog for 22 minutes when you get home. It's something you can do for the rest of your life without feeling overwhelmed. (And for those of you who are up for it, feel free to make those 44 minutes an intense boot camp or spin class—I'm certainly not stopping you. Whatever your fitness goals, you should focus on challenging yourself without getting burned out.)

There are lots of other simple ways to ratchet up your daily dose of physical activity. Here are some easy suggestions to help you to avoid the sedentary lifestyle:

- Take stairs rather than the elevator or escalator whenever you can.

- After lunch and dinner, walk around the block.

- When you find yourself talking to a friend on your cell, put in an earpiece and walk around your neighborhood.

- Get a long-corded or wireless headset if you use a landline in your office. (Or take calls on your cell.) When you're on calls, just stand or pace.

- When you're watching TV, walk around during commercials. You could even hula hoop, hold the plank position, or do crunches!

- Consider a standing-height desk, or an exercise ball to sit on at your office, and alternate sitting on a chair and the ball. Sitting on a ball engages core muscles and burns more energy.

- Park far away from your office or grocery store. Make a habit of choosing the least convenient spot in the lot.

- If you take public transportation, get off a stop early and make up the difference on foot.

- Rescue an animal. Owning a dog makes frequent walks nonnegotiable! (The companionship and unconditional love are big bonuses, too.)

Once you start moving more, you will quickly find that your whole life has improved, including your sleep habits, another essential element of thinking and feeling better.

# CHAPTER 10

# Light, Sleep, and Technology

"I'm a total night owl," Peter announced proudly. "I'm never asleep before three A.M., and I'd guess that I pull all-nighters at least three or four times a week. Comes in really handy, too, given how many times I have to talk to folks in India or China or wherever. But I'm lucky because I've always been a night person."

A website developer in his early 40s, Peter was a shy man who had come to me for problems he couldn't quite put his finger on. He had a wide circle of friends, but he still felt lonely. He was in a long-term relationship, but he wasn't completely satisfied, either sexually or on a purely emotional level. He tried to live a healthy life and exercise, but he had started to put on weight, and he often felt listless and fatigued.

"I feel like everything is in shades of gray," he told me. "Everything is just okay—but not great. And I'm just okay, too—not full of great ideas and creativity and whatnot, just kind of coasting along. I don't know how I got like this. And I don't know how to fix it."

Peter's diet sounded healthy when he described it to me, and his workout regimen passed muster, too. It wasn't until he shared his sleeping patterns that I began to suspect where his brain chemistry was running into trouble.

What Peter didn't realize was that sleep plays a huge role in our brain chemistry on multiple levels. Sleep boosts learning and creativity, and acts as the brain's "self-cleaning" cycle to prevent brain fog and get rid of Alzheimer's-causing plaques. And since sleep affects the stress hormone cortisol, it's also involved in weight loss. (Excess cortisol signals the brain to store belly fat, and lack of sleep also triggers a release of hormones that trigger cravings for the unhealthiest foods. Excess cortisol can also negatively affect serotonin and dopamine in the brain.) All of these factors work together in a delicate dance that can be thrown off by just one or two sleepless nights. Is it any wonder there's such a strong relationship between insomnia and depression?

Nature intended for us to sleep at night and be awake during the day. Those of us who, like Peter, work late into the night are challenging our brain chemistry by disregarding our circadian rhythms—our body's natural 24-hour clock. Although I understood why Peter was attached to his late-night cycle, I couldn't help suspecting that both insufficient sleep and disrupted circadian rhythms were contributing to his low-grade depression and his lack of enjoyment in life.

He is like far too many of us in his unnatural relationship with sleep. You know how it goes: either you're unable to fall asleep, or unable to wake up, unable to sleep deeply, or unable to sleep at the right times. All of these increasingly common problems have a bearing on how clearly we think and how alert and positive we feel.

## 24 HOURS OF LIGHT

The pineal glands in our brains produce a hormone called melatonin, which helps regulate our sleeping and waking cycles. When it's dark out, the pineal gland releases more melatonin to signal that it's time for us to wind down and go to sleep. When the first light of morning breaks outside our window, the pineal gland slows down melatonin production, signaling that it's time to wake up.

That's how our bodies are *supposed* to work: a precise mixture of light and dark syncing with our bodies' sleeping and waking cycles, which also involves the suprachiasmatic nucleus (SCN) in the hypothalamus. The SCN synchronizes the body's sleep-wake cycle with the light-dark cycle of the environment and regulates our personal circadian rhythms, which are likely to be close to—but not exactly—24 hours. (Circadian rhythms don't just affect our sleep cycles but our entire bodies, even our DNA. In one 2013 study, subjects' blood samples revealed that just one week of insufficient sleep affected over 700 genes.[1])

Light is the great equalizer that allows us to live, work, and play on roughly the same schedule. But suddenly there's too much of it, and our bodies just can't cope. These days, we are surrounded by light *all the time*. It's not just the glow from skyscrapers so massive that they're visible from space. It's the tiny lights of our iPhones and tablets that we check constantly, even when we're lying in bed.

Over the past decades, even the *color* of the light has changed from the ambient red glow of an Edison bulb or a 60-watt incandescent to the predominantly blue light of compact fluorescent bulbs, LEDs, and the electronic screens of laptops, TVs, iPhones, and iPads. All of these devices emit more blue light, and blue light—along with genuine full-spectrum sunshine—is particularly good at suppressing melatonin production in our brains. All of this light around the clock means that our bodies no longer know when they're supposed to be asleep.

In the world before electricity, many people spent over 12 hours every day in darkness—or even more in some places and at certain times of the year—meaning the pineal gland released elevated levels of melatonin for half of every day. When's the last time you went 12 continuous hours with no light . . . or no iPhone?

## HOW MUCH SLEEP IS ENOUGH?

Another problem with checking all that technology at night: you might end up staying up later in the evening and sleeping later in the morning, meaning you'll miss the time of day with the most healing concentration of full-spectrum sunlight.[2] Exposing yourself to light in the morning is just as important as avoiding it in the evening. Daytime exposure to sunlight gives you a little boost of vitamin D while signaling your brain to sync rhythms associated with energy and mood.

Unfortunately, the vast majority of us aren't getting that necessary light. We spend our days inside buildings, often far from windows. And most indoor lighting isn't bright enough to give the brain strong enough signals to affect circadian rhythms.

Our lifestyles are profoundly undermining our bodies' natural rhythms: our days are dark when they should be light, and our nights are bright blue when they should be black. This disruption in circadian rhythms can do two things. First, it keeps us up too late. For most of us, this means we don't sleep enough. Second, our bodies don't know when it's time to wake up. So for others, it results in sleeping too much. Both too much and too little sleep are detrimental to mind and body.

The average American is sleeping almost an hour less than just a generation ago. Our constantly connected, smartphone-tethered ways may have some bearing on Americans getting an average of six and a half hours of sleep on weeknights, which is less sleep than all but one of the other countries surveyed in a major poll. American women fared especially poorly, with 67 percent reporting having trouble sleeping multiple times a week.

But even though 73 percent of Americans who don't get enough sleep *know* how their sleep habits are damaging their health, the majority of us use an electronic gadget in the hour before bed. Perhaps that's because not enough of us realize how this constant exposure to light is affecting our sleep—or how dangerous it is to be even moderately sleep deprived.

Did you know that driving on little sleep can be as bad as—or even worse than—driving drunk because many under-rested people don't even know they're impaired? Research shows that being awake for 21 hours is the equivalent of having a blood alcohol level of .08.[3] And scarily, a AAA survey found that 40 percent of drivers report falling asleep or nodding off while driving; more than 25 percent report driving while they were so tired that they had trouble keeping their eyes open.

So what's the magic number when it comes to sleep? Six hours might *seem* like a reasonable amount of shut-eye, but a University of Pennsylvania experiment found that people who slept about six hours for multiple nights in a row had the same performance deficits as subjects who had been totally deprived of sleep for two nights.[4] Even more alarming is that when the subjects were asked to report their subjective experience of sleepiness throughout the study, they were largely unaware of the deficits.

That's because, unfortunately, chronic sleep deprivation has become our new normal. We're so used to being a little tired all the time that we think we're fine when we're anything but. Think about how serious the consequences might be: even a slightly delayed reaction time could mean the difference between hitting the brakes at the right moment and smashing into the car in front of you.

Research also shows that it doesn't take two weeks of sleep deprivation to lead to more car accidents. It happens in just *one night* with just *one hour* of tinkering with our delicate sleep-wake cycle. The proof: there is usually a spike in car accidents the Monday after daylight savings.[5]

So don't fool yourself: getting six hours of sleep simply isn't enough. A good night's sleep is roughly eight hours. Anything less just won't cut it.

## SLEEP, MOOD, AND MEMORY

Getting enough sleep won't just improve your alertness levels. It will improve your mood, too. When you don't sleep enough, your levels of stress hormones like cortisol go up. And when stress hormones go up, dopamine levels go down. Low dopamine levels will leave you feeling unhappy, unmotivated, and unfocused—a perfect recipe for depression. Chronically high cortisol levels have also been shown to prevent serotonin from binding in several areas of the brain, which also contributes to increased anxiety.[6]

*Too little sleep → more cortisol → more stress → low dopamine →
chronic depression*

Sleep also supports learning and neurogenesis, strengthening neural connections and consolidating memories that you encoded during the day, which allows short-term memories to become long-term ones.

So even if you're one of those people who *think* they perform well with just five or six hours of sleep, you're bypassing a crucial step in the fight against brain fog: activating your brain's so-called wash cycle. A 2013 animal study showed that during sleep, channels between neurons expand up to 60 percent, which allows cerebrospinal fluid in. All that extra space between neurons is your brain getting ready to get hosed down: the cerebrospinal fluid flushes out the Alzheimer's disease-causing plaques. This "wash cycle" is much more effective when you're asleep, which means more "junk" gets cleared from your brain.[7]

That's why it came as no surprise when another study found that mice who sleep for only four hours a day had more Alzheimer's-causing plaques in the brain.[8] Sleep might also reinforce brain cells; a 2013 study showed that while mice slept, their brains were making more myelin, the brain cells' insulation that allows the electrical current of happiness to flow freely.[9]

## OTHER HEALTH CONSEQUENCES OF INSUFFICIENT SLEEP

If you're chronically underrested, you're more likely to gain weight. The reason for this is that circadian rhythms don't just make you sleep: they also affect your metabolism and energy levels. In one study, exposure to light early in the morning—when blue light is at its highest level—has been linked to a lower body mass index. The earlier the exposure to light, the leaner the subjects tended to be. The researchers conducting this study found that daytime light exposure needs to be at a level that is difficult to achieve with indoor lighting.[10]

Levels of leptin, the hormone that makes you feel full after eating, go down when circadian rhythms are disturbed. The result is that you'll probably eat more and have higher blood sugar, which, as we've seen, can lead to diabetes, brain fog, and dementia. All of these factors are endlessly connected.

*Too little sleep → Not enough leptin → More overeating → Higher blood sugar → weight gain → possibility of developing diabetes, brain fog, and dementia*

Proper melatonin levels are also important for staying healthy. Melatonin—which, again, is a hormone produced by the pineal gland that helps regulate sleeping and waking cycles—doesn't just help you sleep; it's also a potent antioxidant. This hormone becomes even more precious with age, since production goes down.

Insufficient melatonin levels are associated with an increased cancer risk. Just take the extreme example of night-shift workers, whose schedules lead to an artificial suppression of melatonin. An analysis of 21 different studies examining night-shift workers revealed up to a 70 percent increased risk of breast cancer in women and a 40 percent increased risk of prostate cancer in men.[11] By contrast, people in low-sunlight areas like Alaska or Greenland (where people tend to have higher levels of melatonin) have low rates of breast and prostate cancer.[12]

## Control Caffeine

Here's another compelling reason to avoid OD'ing on caffeine: when you ignore nature's pattern by staying up all night because you're buzzed from caffeine, you suppress the release of melatonin from your pineal gland. And, as we've learned, melatonin is not just a "sleep hormone." It's also a potent antioxidant that suppresses cancer and tumor formation in the body.

*Too much caffeine → staying up too late → lower melatonin levels → more cancer → more death.*

To make matters even more complicated, melatonin suppression may be a risk factor for cancer, and cancer itself may depress melatonin production, which increases the risk of the cancer progressing.[13] No wonder a review of several studies that included over 1 million people found that people who sleep either too little or too much face a greater risk of death.[14]

## PRESSING THE OVERRIDE BUTTON

But what if you *just can't sleep?* Trust me—we've all been there. A reported 50 to 70 million Americans struggle with chronic sleep disorders.[15] And according to the CDC, roughly that same number of Americans—at least 50 million—report an insufficient amount of sleep.

Unfortunately, rather than get their body's natural rhythms back in order, many of these people choose to press the proverbial "override button" by taking a prescription sleep aid, which can knock them out regardless of where they are in their circadian cycles. To judge by the sales of the number-one prescription sleeping pill in the country, Ambien, lots and lots of people are going this route.

The numbers are truly shocking. The company that makes Ambien reported *12 billion* of these pills have been swallowed between 1988 and 2006.[16] In 2012, Ambien was the twelfth most prescribed medication in the country, and the second most prescribed psychiatric medication, with over 44 million prescriptions filled.[17]

People are so desperate for a good night's sleep that they ignore the increasingly alarming headlines about the drug's dangers. The crash of the Staten Island ferry in 2003, which killed 11 people, may have been linked to Ambien.[18] In 2007, a Sydney man who jumped to his death from a high-rise balcony may have been sleepwalking while on Ambien.[19]

There have also been plenty of reports about the dangers of driving while on Ambien. In 2006, Patrick Kennedy crashed his car while

Ambien was in his system. A toxicologist found 187 drivers who had been arrested in Wisconsin over a five-year period had Ambien in their blood.[20] A 2008 study in Miami found that 5 percent of drivers pulled over and screened for a DUI had Ambien in their system.[21]

Even if you take the medication as prescribed, get a good night's sleep, and wake up after eight hours, driving might still be dangerous, especially if you're female, since men metabolize Ambien much more quickly than women. In 2013, the FDA recommended lower doses of Ambien for women after studies showed that 15 percent of women still had enough Ambien in their blood to impair their driving eight hours after taking the non–extended release 10 mg dose. For the newer extended-release Ambien, that number jumps to 33 percent of women.[22] Ambien is also problematic for seniors, since cognitive impairment and falls can result. Research shows for people over 60, the benefit of the medication probably does not outweigh the risk.[23]

According to the U.S. Substance Abuse and Mental Health Services Administration, Ambien comes with other dangers, too. ER visits for adverse reactions to Ambien climbed 220 percent from 2005 to 2010. Most were women, and the most common age group was 45 to 65.[24] Researchers also identified an association between Ambien and both cancer and death in 2012, though they couldn't conclude that the relationship was a cause-and-effect one.[25] Still, shouldn't we be more wary before indiscriminately popping these and other sleeping pills on a regular basis? In a recent New Yorker interview, a researcher who examined the electronic health records of more than 30,000 people to study the relationship between Ambien and death said, "My best estimate is that drugs like zolpidem (Ambien) are killing as many people as cigarettes."[26]

Ambien might also leave people thinking and feeling worse. Anterograde amnesia—which leads to an inability to remember the recent past—is another extremely troubling possible side effect for what might be as many as 5 percent of users.[27] Some people, after taking the drug, may binge eat or even have sex with no memory of the event, which is why Ambien has reportedly been used as a date-rape drug.[28]

Even without these frightening potential outcomes, Ambien still isn't all that effective at tackling insomnia. Rebound insomnia often occurs, meaning once you stop taking Ambien, your insomnia is actually worse than it was before you started taking a sleeping pill.[29]

Pressing the override button is *not* the answer. As with all the other psychiatric medications we've discussed, there are just too many risks involved for you to take these medications without first investigating other options. If you're determined to remake your relationship with sleep, start by committing to some lifestyle adjustments to get your days (and nights!) back in order with your natural rhythms. It might take more effort than popping another pill, but the results will last far longer, and will leave you feeling better than you have in years.

## ACTION PLAN

If you suffer from insomnia, I really encourage you to try a drug-free option first, starting with cognitive behavioral therapy, which has been shown to help people fall asleep faster than prescription sleeping pills do.[30]

Small changes in diet can be extremely effective as well, since most Americans aren't getting enough omega-3s, which are essential for supporting melatonin production. The omega-3 DHA found in seafood has been shown to improve sleep duration and quality. In the 7-Day Mood Revolution, you'll be eating one DHA-rich omega-3 superfood per day, which may help you sleep better naturally.

If you still need some help going to sleep, time-release melatonin supplements can be an effective option. You can find these pills over the counter at pretty much any drugstore.[31] But opt for the smaller doses like the 1 mg time-release version, since too much can also disrupt your natural sleep-wake cycle. Melatonin is useful for people with insomnia because research shows they're likely to have lower levels of melatonin than people without insomnia.[32] (And since melatonin production decreases as you age, insomnia is likely to get worse as the years pass.)

One study showed that melatonin can reduce the amount of time it takes to fall asleep; in some cases, the supplements actually outperformed some prescription sleep aids.[33] Melatonin can also promote both sleep quality and morning alertness, which can be especially helpful for two groups of people who have been shown to experience significant dangers when taking Ambien: women and the elderly.[34] And unlike prescription sleep aids, melatonin comes with no withdrawal effects. That said, while melatonin can correct your body's circadian rhythms, too much can throw them off. Our bodies produce only about 0.3 mg per day, so start with the lowest dose you need to help improve sleep. And, as always, inform your doctor of any medications or supplements before you take them.

## OTHER SOLUTIONS

**Soak Up Some Sunshine:** Expose your eyes to light first thing in the morning by opening your blinds and turning on your lights as soon as you wake up. Take a walk outside in the morning and over your lunch hour—you'll get exercise and healing light at the same time. If you have a window in your office, position your desk so that you face it, or are at least perpendicular to the window.

**Rethink Your Lighting:** If you're stuck in a windowless office all morning, invest in the LED light bulbs created by Definity Digital. Their "Awake and Alert" light bulb produces blue light to keep you awake, and it's bright enough to help affect sleep-wake cycles. You can also use a special bulb like Definity Digital's "Good Night" light bulb, which filters out the blue light in the afternoon and evening, when it's best to avoid fluorescent and LED lighting. Both bulbs, however, emit light that looks like a regular light bulb. While they're more expensive than traditional light bulbs, Definity's lights are very energy efficient, using only about 10 watts to replace 60-watt bulbs. Another bonus: they last much longer than either incandescent or fluorescent bulbs. In rooms with fluorescent lighting like the kitchen, consider installing a light-detecting night-light so you don't need to turn on the lights in the evening. Install dimmers on your lights. At night, use incandescent lights on a dim setting.

**Nap When Needed**: If you benefit from naps to stay alert and strong, by all means take them. Research shows that naps can improve performance even if the quality of sleep during naps isn't great. One study showed that just 18 minutes of sleep provided improvements in reaction time for air traffic controllers. You may need to set aside about 40 minutes, however, as it may take about 20 minutes to actually fall asleep.[35] Since your sleep-wake cycle tends to dip after lunch, the best time for a short nap is probably in the midafternoon. Keep it short to prevent it from interfering with your nighttime rhythms. Scheduling your naps in advance is another good strategy, as it allows your brain to prepare for this ritual, and you may find it easier to fall asleep for a restorative rest. You can and should even nap on the road if necessary: if you find yourself sleepy on a long drive, pull over for about a half hour in a safe place and rest.

**Reform Your Evening Relationship with Electronics**: We will go into this recommendation in more detail in the following chapter, but if you're having trouble sleeping, you should make every effort to avoid electronics, especially TVs and cell phones, in the evenings. It's a good idea to turn off all devices three hours before bedtime. (Just imagine what this abstinence will do for your connections with your loved ones!) If you must remain plugged in, turn your phone, tablet, or laptop to the dimmest setting possible, or—even better—use them while wearing sunglasses with orange-tinted lenses, which can block the blue light that can alter your circadian rhythms. Remove TVs and other electronic devices from your bedroom. Instead of charging your phone in your bedroom, place it in the living room or kitchen to avoid nighttime checking. If you read before bed, ditch your electronic reader and instead read old-fashioned bound books with dim lighting.

**Check Your Temperature**: High-quality sleep isn't just affected by the brightness or color of light but by body temperature. Because body temperature fluctuates during the day and night, room temperature should also vary. Your body temperature is higher in the afternoon and evening, then starts to dip when it's time for bed, and reaches its lowest in the morning hours when some of the most restorative sleep is taking place. Keeping your room cool can help facilitate this natural cooling process that occurs during sleep. While 70 degrees is a good room temperature while you're awake, a good sleeping room temperature should be even lower, somewhere around 66 to 68 degrees. Another idea is to take a hot shower or bath before bed, which can help induce sleep for two reasons: the warm water will relax your muscles and when you get out of the shower or bath, your body temperature will dip. For the best sleep, keep your body as cool as possible, with the exception of your feet. Make sure they're warm, wearing socks if you need to, as having cold feet may prevent you from falling asleep.

CHAPTER 11

# DIGITAL DISTRACTION

Monica's problem was evident to me from the first 90 seconds of our session. Armed with a BlackBerry for work e-mails and an iPhone for personal calls and texts, she kept both on when she sat down. She was a mom, a high-powered publicist—and constantly connected. She had to be! She was always waiting for that emergency call, e-mail, or text to come in. In reality, the constant pings weren't emergencies, but rather reminders about meetings from her assistant, press release approval requests, and messages about a client's dress being panned at an awards show the night before.

Monica's nonstop barrage of calls, texts, Tweets, and e-mails had left her in a state of constant distraction. She always felt only "half there," never fully engaged in the present moment. What's worse, her perpetual distractedness was beginning to erode her relationship with her husband and kids. Her resulting symptoms were a mixed bag: a little anxiety, a little insomnia, a little depression.

As Monica described the stresses of trying to juggle a marriage, motherhood, and a high-stress job, she teared up when she remembered her nine-year-old daughter sighing and saying, "Mommy, you never look at me when I'm talking to you. You love working more than you love me."

That comment was Monica's tipping point. She was ready and willing to turn her life around.

"Dr. Mike, my daughter helped me realize that I'm never going to get back these moments with my kids. I need your help to reprioritize my life, but frankly, I'm a little scared because I'm not sure if it's even possible. I feel like I need every day to be thirty hours to get everything done."

"While I can't make the actual day longer," I said, "I can certainly help you to become more present, which *will* actually buy you precious minutes and hours each and every day."

I explained that while most people assume multitasking saves time, the opposite is actually true. Mindfully "single-tasking" won't just help you feel less frantic and more focused; it will also help you become more efficient so you can finish that press release, spreadsheet, or memo more quickly. You can even use social media and browse the Internet mindfully instead of just mindlessly procrastinating on the computer all day.

When you're more focused on work tasks, you'll have more time left over to give to things that are important to you—like quality time with your family. And when you give your time to the people you care about, you'll be truly present, and presence is one of the most magical and transformative gifts one human being can give to another. It can make or break a marriage or friendship. It can make your child feel seen and heard—as opposed to unimportant and unloved.

"It won't happen overnight, Monica. But I promise you that if you are willing to make some simple changes, your life will improve dramatically."

## DISTRACTED ALL DAY AND NIGHT

Does Monica's predicament sound familiar to you? Have you ever wasted a morning at work checking and refreshing all your devices—only to find out that you've gotten no work done?

Here's an all-too-typical scenario: You start off working on a spreadsheet, but suddenly your phone lights up with a text, then a Facebook notification from yet another person who liked that photo you posted last night, followed shortly by a push notification with a breaking news alert. Oh, and there's an Evite for a cocktail party two weeks from now, and then your work phone rings, and then your assistant comes into your office to remind you about the half-dozen meetings and conference calls you have on the schedule today. Shoot! You'd totally forgotten almost half of them.

*Man, I'm so scatterbrained,* you think. You clearly need some coffee. You chat with a friend for 15 minutes in the break room, half listening and half mentally listing all the things you should be getting done instead. You return to your office, and in the hour that elapsed since you got to work you could have finished that spreadsheet. Now you're freaking out because your first of many meetings starts in ten minutes, which means you'll have to take the spreadsheet home and finish it in the evening. *Oh well,* you think; *I'll just do it in front of the TV while eating dinner and trying to catch up with my boyfriend about his day.*

You finally finish the spreadsheet at 1 A.M. A few hours after you stumble exhausted into work the next day, your boss sends you a not-all-that-nice e-mail pointing out several errors you made in the document. By this point you feel totally overwhelmed. You're even more behind, since you now have to correct yesterday's work while also finishing today's.

When you consider how accustomed most of us have gotten to distraction, is it any wonder ADHD rates are skyrocketing? They have tripled in children, and with broader diagnostic requirements for adult ADHD, the already-through-the-roof adult ADHD rates are likely to spike as well. But while Adderall can improve attention for most—and is absolutely necessary for some—it's not the only solution to our inattentiveness issue. Turning off your ringer or blocking your access to Facebook for an hour can have the same effect.

It's worth making these small but meaningful changes, because digital distraction doesn't just make us feel scattered; it's killing people. One study showed that driving while using a phone is comparable to drunk driving.[1] From 2005 to 2010, the number of pedestrians who were struck and killed by distracted drivers rose 50 percent in the U.S. Distracted *walking* has even become a problem. Yes, that's right: people cannot even look both ways before they cross the street because they're too busy staring at their phones.

You can almost understand the lure of the phone when you're stuck in traffic for 90 minutes, but we're now so addicted to our phones that we're sucking all the simple joy out of a five-minute walk.

One thing to understand about our phones and computers is that all the blinking lights, dings, and dynamic ads scrolling across the screen when we're trying to read the news give our brains a tiny hit of dopamine. It's not dissimilar to the way dopamine surges through the brain of a compulsive gambler when he's sitting in front of the slot machine. Facebook likes, Twitter retweets, Snapchat pics, Instagram followers, and Tinder matches have started to exert an addictive pull on us. A little is never enough: we have become dependent on that little surge of pleasure that pulses through us every time someone likes one of our status updates, so we do it again and again and again.

## MULTITASKING MANIA

We are even scattered and inattentive during our leisure activities. According to a recent survey, 61 percent of people watch TV and browse the Internet simultaneously—we can't even focus during our downtime!

But in reality, what's called "multitasking" is really just rapid single-tasking. A 2009 study showed that subjects trained to do two things simultaneously did indeed increase the speed of processing and therefore got better at "multitasking"—or so it appeared. But brain scans revealed that while it appeared the subjects were multitasking, they were really switching between tasks so rapidly that it gave the *illusion* of doing two things simultaneously.[2]

And while we are constantly switching between tasks, we are wasting precious time. One 2001 study showed that as the complexity of tasks grew, subjects began to waste more time switching between them. Multiplication and division, for example, lead to more lost time than addition. The real-world translation is that you probably won't lose much time chatting with your spouse about your day while doing the dishes, but you *will* start to suffer when responding to an important e-mail while simultaneously discussing your daughter's recent behavior problems with your spouse.

The study also found that multitasking led to subjects' brains becoming overloaded, so they couldn't filter out irrelevant information.[3] They would've been more efficient giving all their attention to one task, finishing it, and then moving onto the next task. The burdens of task switching can lead to a *40 percent decrease* in efficiency. Can you imagine how much more time you would have if you were 40 percent more efficient?

Another study specifically examined the performance and memory of "heavy" versus "light" media multitaskers. While you'd think those who identify as "heavy media multitaskers" would be better at filtering out irrelevant stimuli and faster at switching between tasks, they were actually *worse* on these measures when compared to light media multitaskers.[4] The results demonstrated that light media multitaskers were better at focusing their attention on a single task since they could filter out irrelevant stimuli from the environment.

So before considering Adderall to treat your difficulty concentrating, try out some mindfulness techniques that will allow you to cut back on multitasking, and become more efficient in the process. Mindfulness—doing one thing at a time and paying attention while doing it—is a powerful antidote to the barrage of distractions that come at us day and night.

Meditation is another simple practice that can help improve focus, and it doesn't take a lot of effort to reap big results. One study showed that meditation improved attention while decreasing fatigue and anxiety with just 20 minutes of practice for five consecutive days.[5] Another study showed that the benefits of meditation were apparent in brain scans and improved subjects' memories with just *12 minutes a day* of practice. That's the amount of time you spend drowsing through commercials during a single 30-minute sitcom![6] In the next section, I will be introducing you to some super-simple, do-anywhere meditation techniques that force you to slow down and pay closer attention to the world around you.

## THE SOCIAL MEDIA CONUNDRUM

Ironically, the very inventions designed to help us to stay con-nected—everything from cell phones to social media—are making us more *disconnected* from the people we love most. The texts we send during dinner distance us from the person we're having dinner with. Constantly taking photos with our phones can make us less present in the moment itself. Facebook status updates have increasingly become "one-ups" that can lead to a bad mood for those who see them. So our social media addictions are not just fraying our attention spans and making us think worse; they're making us *feel* worse, too.

So it's time to examine your social media use. Ask yourself: is my social media use improving my real-life relationships, or is it replacing them? If you use Facebook to stay connected to good friends in other states or make plans with local ones, that's great. But if you spend two hours a night studying the vacation photos of someone you barely know (and feeling depressed by how much less glamorous your own life is in comparison), you might want to consider devoting that time to meeting up with a friend for a post-work tea or dinner instead. The other question to ask yourself is: *Why* am I going on social media right now? Am I doing it to procrastinate? Am I doing it to "Facebook stalk" my ex, which will depress me and prevent me from moving on with my love life?[7] Am I doing it because it's less demanding than picking up the phone and making plans with a friend? This type of self-examination shows how even social media use can start to take on a mindful quality.

And speaking of all those Instagram and Facebook photos, why are *you* posting so many? If you think you're capturing a moment to imprint it deeper in your memory, research shows that the act of taking the photo might actually make the moment *less* memorable.[8] Now, this isn't to say that you shouldn't take pictures. But for the digitally distracted, compelled-to-photograph-and-post-every-single-waking-moment types, it's probably best to rein in the obsession. Enjoy the aroma of that coffee and the company of friends without giving in to the compulsion to catalog the experience. Just be there and make full contact with the present moment without a camera coming between you and what you're experiencing. Take it all in sans filter. Maybe one day you can even graduate to going out to dinner *without* your phone.

And interestingly, by posting fewer pictures of your life, you may actually help your friends feel better about theirs. One recent study showed that subjects felt more negative emotions after going on Facebook. Envy and loneliness may be the result of comparing your own life to an idealized version of others'.[9]

## ACTION PLAN

So as you can see, stepping back from your digital world a bit can be very healthy. But it can also be very hard. At least in the beginning, you might have to take some extreme steps to wean yourself. Here are some great places to start.

**Get an Internet Blocker:** Try out an Internet blocker like mindful-browsing.com, which allows you to block the sites you use to waste time. For the truly committed (who also happen to be Mac users), there's also selfcontrolapp.com, which will block the sites you choose for a set amount of time, even if you restart your computer. The Freedom Internet blocker, which you can download onto your computer for $10, will disable your Internet connection for up to eight hours. Try using one of these programs for a few minutes at the beginning of the day so you can focus your mind and get into a good work groove.

**Put Some Space Between You and Your Phone:** Whenever you're working, turn off your phone or its ringer. Move the charger from the bedroom to your kitchen or entryway so that you aren't constantly checking your phone instead of going to sleep. And block push notifications so that every single Tweet or Instagram like or *New York Times* notification doesn't interrupt important e-mails or calls. When you get in the car, throw your phone in the trunk or turn off the ringer. There are useful apps that will disable your phone while in motion on both iPhones and Android devices. Try to have one full day of the weekend completely phone free.

**Be More Mindful:** Finding mindfulness, incorporating some of the 12-minute meditation practices that I introduce on pages 219 to 233 into your everyday routine, and decreasing digital distractions can help you lead a more productive and creative life. Without constant technological distractions, even normal acts like daydreaming can become mindful. You can use these moments to toy with new ideas or make future plans—but only if you're alert enough to catch the great ideas as they drift through your head. The 7-Day Spirit Revolution is designed to tackle the attention deficits that patients like Monica—and far too many of us—experience all too frequently.

CHAPTER 12

# An Epidemic of Loneliness

Shannon was a 40-year-old woman with an Ivy League education and a long track record of off-the-charts professional accomplishment. Originally from New York, she had moved to Los Angeles five years earlier to accept a prestigious job. The pencil skirt, red-soled heels, and expensive bag were all visual evidence of her success.

While she was extremely proud of her career, Shannon's single-minded focus on work left little time for socializing or dating. One by one, her friends were getting married and having kids. When she went over to their houses, Shannon—often the only single woman with no kids present—began to feel anxious that she would never find someone to date. These anxieties worsened when she turned 40. Shannon found herself refusing more and more social invitations and felt increasingly isolated from her friends.

Lately, Shannon had also noticed that her one glass of cabernet on weeknights was frequently turning into three. When things were going well at work, she felt in control. When they weren't, she lashed out at her assistant. More and more often, she would go home feeling overwhelmed and exhausted. She started popping a few more Xanax than usual and needed Ambien to sleep most nights.

Underneath the drinking, self-medication, and anxiety, Shannon had one root problem: loneliness. Her family was across the country. She hated being set up and had sworn off online dating after one bad experience.

"Dr. Mike, I just feel so 'over it' these days. The littlest things are setting me off. I screamed at one of the managers who reports to me for something that wasn't that big a deal. I used to have tons of friends, but now they're all married with kids. Do I have to choose between having a career and having a life? That's how it feels to me most days. And this is awful to admit, but if I see one more adorable baby photo on Facebook, I'm going to lose it."

I listened and said something very simple: "Shannon, you sound so lonely."

With that one sentence, she began to cry.

I continued: "And I believe your anger and sadness are telling you that something in your life needs to change."

"I know," she said in a voice completely unlike her usually assertive tone.

"I bet it's quite rare that you let people see this soft, vulnerable part of you that I'm seeing right now. And I wonder if that's part of the problem."

"Probably," she said. "But what am I supposed to do? Crying isn't going to change anything."

"You're right. The first step is what you just did: acknowledging what exactly is making you so 'over it,' which is your loneliness. Instead of you self-medicating or withdrawing from your friends, you and I are going to figure out what changes you need to make in your life. Right now, you've got all your eggs in the 'work' basket, so it's no wonder you get so angry at the little things at work, because when that's all you've got, you *really* need that one thing to go well."

In my work with Shannon, I helped her to look at the relationships she *already* had while starting to cultivate new ones. I prescribed a miracle treatment that has life-altering benefits: connection. We started to change her life one step at a time, beginning with simple things like picking up the phone and calling a friend to have dinner. Instead of spending excess cash on a new pair of $500 shoes, she splurged on a catered dinner party for her friends. For a few months she dated a guy she had met at a friend's kid's party—exactly the type of event she would've sulked through before.

When she started to change her priorities by changing her *actions*, her *thoughts* and *feelings* changed, too. Shannon began to feel happier and more connected to those around her, which made her want to connect even more. She was engaging more with friends and family, and she had made a fair number of new friends, too. About a year later, she actually got engaged to a guy she met online.

She didn't have to quit her job. She didn't have to choose between being a businesswoman and having close relationships. I'm here to tell you: if you want it all, you really can have it all. It just requires some conscious effort, a little faith, and a willingness to change so you can cultivate balance in your life.

## STRANGERS IN STRANGE LANDS

Current trends in our country are putting more and more people at risk for loneliness. Whenever I meet new people here in Los Angeles, I inevitably ask where they're from—and I can't help but notice that the answer is almost never Los Angeles. It seems as if almost everyone has recently moved here from some other city. And this hypermobility is happening all over the country.

In generations past, many people stayed with the same company for their entire career. This is now quite rare, and the globalized economy often requires that people make geographical decisions based on where the next promotion is—or where there's any job at all. It is now common to not know, talk to, or even make eye contact with neighbors. Many people have a thousand Facebook friends but very few high-quality, face-to-face relationships.

According to the U.S. Census Bureau, the number of Americans living alone has tripled since 1970, and the number of households consisting of a married couple living with children has been cut in half. People are waiting longer to get married, and those marriages are less likely to last than in generations past. People are also living longer, which means more widows and widowers, and research shows the majority of these people are uninterested in remarriage.

Those in small, rural towns are likely to have children and grandchildren who have left for larger, urban areas. While there are many benefits to these social trends, like a greater variety of career options, there is also much more loneliness, which can have effects that are more devastating than many people realize.

The link between loneliness and depression is reciprocal. Loneliness has been shown to be associated with depressive symptoms.[1] And, of course, people who are depressed are more likely to isolate themselves, which leads to even more loneliness—the conditions reinforce each other in a downward spiral.

Paradoxically, the antidepressant treatment more and more Americans resort to when they're feeling lonely may worsen the problem. A 2009 study looked at the relationship between SSRI antidepressants and what's known as "emotional blunting."[2] The majority of subjects reported feeling dulled, numbed, or flat with general reductions in positive emotions, which they attributed to the antidepressant. But the most disturbing finding is how this blunting affected their ability to connect to others. Many felt detached from the people in their lives, including their significant other, children, family, and friends.

I've already said that SSRIs can be essential when it comes to treating clinical and potentially life-threatening depression, but in many other instances, they can hurt more than they help. Popping a pill won't help if the root of your problem is that you need to meet somebody and fall in love. One celebrated researcher who has conducted studies using brain scans of the progression of love in the human brain has suggested that SSRIs may prevent people from falling in love. When people first fall in love, dopamine soars while serotonin dips. As a result, you feel excited, turned on . . . and also anxious and obsessed with your love object, which may help cement a strong bond. You stay up all night talking about life. You want to be in physical contact at all times. But if SSRIs block this dip in serotonin, this obsessive quality associated with falling in love may not happen. Potential passion could end up being more "take it or leave it."

Loneliness and anxiety also go hand in hand, as perceived isolation can make us view the world as more dangerous.[3] This distorted perspective might lead us to filter experiences through a mantra of "I'm not okay" or "I'm not safe." This leads to a hypervigilance in your daily activities that can result in low serotonin and high stress hormones. This neurological state will leave many wanting to self-medicate with a Xanax and/or three glasses of wine, but this is no long-term solution. It's far more healing to pick up the phone and go out to dinner or a movie with an old friend.

## BUILDING RELATIONSHIPS

The link between loneliness and depression might not surprise you, but what about the connection between loneliness and mortality? A review of 148 studies that included more than 300,000 people suggested that extreme loneliness may actually be deadlier than smoking and *twice as deadly* as obesity. In this analysis, stronger social relationships resulted in a 50 percent increased likelihood of survival.[4] No wonder social connectedness has been called a "behavioral vaccine."[5]

The lesson here is that human beings have an innate need to feel supported, connected, and loved. This is not strictly a psychological need, because psychological needs affect physical health and vice versa. If we can get surgeon general warnings on cigarette boxes, maybe we should also broadcast public service announcements to the tune of, "Hey, you, eating takeout on the couch and watching TV by yourself again. Call somebody. Make plans. Join a club. Being alone all the time is extremely hazardous to your health!"

No wonder one of the best predictors of feeling better is being married, since it guarantees that we won't be alone when we come home from work or when we're in a particularly stressful situation. According to the National Opinion Research Center's General Social Survey of over 40,000 people, about 40 percent of married people rated themselves as being "very happy" compared to only about 20 percent of never married, separated, or divorced people.

But don't be in a hurry to marry just anybody, because people in not very happy marriages are also not very happy people, with a dismal 3 percent rating themselves as "very happy." But we *should* aspire to cultivate a healthy union with a person we respect and admire, because married people who rated their marriages as "very happy" are also *by far* the happiest in their lives.[6]

It's not just the relationship but the frequent expression of love that helps people feel better and live longer. In one long-term study, men who had sex at least twice a week were much less likely to die from a heart attack compared to those who had less sex.[7] Could more sex with one's significant other be an effective heart disease prevention strategy? What a great idea: it's free, has no side effects, and it's also a good deal more enjoyable than popping another pill. (And speaking of pills and sex, one of the most common side effects of SSRIs is the sexual dysfunction that 83 percent of patients reported experiencing in one study—a condition that can, of course, inhibit connection and intimacy.)[8]

Whether or not you ever get married, it's indisputable that cultivating connection, support, and companionship is a nonnegotiable for thinking and feeling better. And no matter how old you are, if you're married, single, or dating, you *always* have an opportunity to connect to others. You may not be able to control when or where you meet the love of your life, but you can certainly control whether you accept that dinner invitation, create that online dating profile, say yes to that blind date, pick up the phone and call your best friend or mom, or even adopt a rescue animal. Oxytocin, the neurotransmitter of cuddling and connection, is released whether you're spooning your significant other, breast-feeding your child, or just rubbing Fido's belly.

The *how* of connection matters as well. Like a well-rounded retirement portfolio, you should diversify your relationships with a combination of romantic love, friendship, and family. As tempting or easy as it may be, don't put all your eggs in one basket. It's vital to cultivate a balance between the relationship with your significant other and other relationships in your life.

The cultural stereotype might be that women desire romantic love more than men, but the reality seems to be that men actually need it more than women. Widows tend to fare better in life than widowers for the simple reason that women are better at maintaining their marriage and strong friendships simultaneously.

When people lose their spouse, remarrying or not remarrying are both suitable options . . . as long as people stay connected. The good news is that as people age (and are more likely to lose their spouse), they are also more likely to socialize with neighbors, volunteer, and attend religious services.[9] So, again, it's not about needing to cohabitate; it's about staying connected to those around you. It's also clear that both the quantity and the quality of your relationships do matter, with the latter carrying more weight.[10]

Speaking of quality versus quantity, you may notice that you do some friend "pruning" as you get older. Your life as a 40-year-old mom with a full-time job is probably busier than it was when you were in high school, so you simply don't have as much time for friendships.

Far more important than the total number of friends you can have is the number of very *close friends* you have. These are confidants, people you can tell anything to. Research shows that most Americans used to have about three of these. It's no wonder iconic shows feature an ensemble cast of four close friends. *Sex and the City's* Carrie had Samantha, Charlotte, and Miranda; *Entourage's* Vincent Chase has E, Johnny Drama, and Turtle. And the *Golden Girls'* Dorothy, Blanche, Ma, and Rose all had one another.

But someone may need to inform Hollywood's television writers that they should start writing one less main character into those scripts, because research shows that the average number of confidants has shrunk from about three in the 1980s to two in the 2000s. And about one in four Americans report having none.[11]

This dynamic is playing out in our virtual worlds as well. In 2009, one survey revealed that only about half of the Facebook users had "pruned" their friends by unfriending somebody. In 2012, that number jumped to two-thirds. It seems that we are all inherently aware, even in our online interactions, that quality trumps quantity.

Even worse than feeling alone in a room by yourself is feeling alone in a room full of people—or even on a Facebook page with thousands of "friends." Social media was supposed to make it easier to keep in touch with friends and enhance connections, but one 2013 study showed that checking Facebook actually made people feel *worse*.[12] Have we reached the tipping point where social media actually *prevents* us from feeling connected to others? Do we stay home more perusing Facebook instead of going out with others and strengthening our own relationships?

Real-life, flesh-and-blood relationships are extremely important both for our emotional health and for our brains. A study of more than 800 older adults over the course of many years showed that being lonely can *double* your risk of Alzheimer's disease in addition to leading to cognitive decline.[13] Feeling connected to others can even help you preserve intelligence over time. One remarkable study that followed almost 500 people over the span of 70 years, measuring subjects' IQ at age 11 and then again at age 79, demonstrated that strong social networks and feeling supported can help preserve cognitive abilities and intelligence over the years.[14]

To reap all these benefits (and get a better social life to boot!), we will be engaging in activities that promote connection and neurogenesis in the 7-Day Energy Revolution. Growing and challenging your brain also means forming new social networks and getting out of the house to stay active and mobile—and, even more important, filling your life with a sense of belonging, connection, and purpose.

## CREATING CONNECTIONS

Try some of these simple suggestions for living a less isolated, and more fulfilling, life:

- Ask a special someone on a date. If you don't have a special someone (yet!), tell your friends you're ready for blind dating, or go ahead and take the plunge and create an online dating profile.

- Be the one to initiate sex tonight.

- Call someone just to say, "I love you."

- Coach a kid's sports team—even if you don't have kids!

- Cuddle with your significant other or pet.

- Host a dinner party.

- Join a free meetup.com group—you can find everything from hiking groups to social organizations designed for meeting new people.

- Plan a vacation with your best friends from high school or college.

- Take a dance class.

# CHAPTER 13

# Spiritual Starvation

John was a successful and seemingly happy businessman, husband, and father of two. On the surface, everything about his life appeared to be exceptional: he made a six-figure income, loved his family and friends, and was in great health. So why had he started therapy with me?

He told me that while he considered himself happy, he had recently started to sense that there was something missing in his life. He had everything he'd ever wanted, so why did he feel an occasional sense of emptiness?

In talking to John, I could tell that for all his warmth, he was a deeply logical person. He was a thinker, not a feeler. He only believed in things that could be scientifically proven. His parents' rigid evangelical Christian beliefs, for example, had never made sense to him, so he hadn't stepped inside a church since high school (except for other people's weddings). It seemed that since his parents' faith wasn't the right fit for him, he had concluded that *no* religion or spirituality would suit him.

John considered this line of thinking sound and rational. But I believe that it's possible to be simultaneously logical *and* emotional, scientific *and* spiritual, and I tried to prove as much to John—and to see whether an infusion of spirituality might improve his full, well-ordered life.

John started with the simple 12-minute meditations I prescribed. He also spent more time in nature, doing mindful walking meditations where he would shut off his phone and just "be"—a state his linear, means-to-an-end-oriented "doing" mind wasn't used to. He even went to a contemporary church service with his wife and kids and was surprised by how much he enjoyed it. He may not have agreed with everything the pastor said, but that was okay. Just having a reflective hour with his family, free of phones and distractions, was a quiet joy in and of itself.

Long after our sessions together had ended, John continued on his own spiritual journey. He wasn't sure *exactly* what he believed in, but he was now invested in the search, and feeling far more fulfilled as a result.

## SEARCHING FOR MEANING

In addition to other trends like living alone, not moving nearly enough, and eating more factory-farmed foods, Americans have become less likely to identify with a religion. According to recent data, one-fifth of Americans don't consider themselves affiliated with any one religion. That number is even higher for Americans under the age of 30, one-third of whom are now religiously unaffiliated.

In the modern, increasingly secular and commercial world, it's becoming easier to forget the profound power spiritual practice exerts over humans. Many people have rejected the religion of their childhood—and replaced it with no spiritual practice at all. This is unfortunate, since age-old spiritual traditions of praying, singing, meditating, and chanting may soothe anxiety even better than prescription medication. The calming music played in many religious services has been shown to improve sleep quality as well.[1]

Finding a spiritual path has been shown to improve happiness levels, too: people who frequently attend religious services are more likely to consider themselves "very happy" and live longer than those who don't.[2] This group might even have lower blood pressure than those who never attend services.[3] One survey showed an association between believing in life after death and lower levels of anxiety and depression—even without attending services.[4]

Of course, you don't have to be affiliated with a specific religion to experience happiness or live a long life. The majority of people who are not affiliated with a religion still believe in God, and many of the unaffiliated still consider themselves to be spiritual or to have a deep connection with nature and the earth.[5] It's also possible to realize some—but not all—of these same benefits by joining a recreational sports team or strengthening friendships.

And people who *do* consider themselves religious but no longer identify with a particular community should start searching for a spiritual home. Try one new service a week for a month. In this day and age, there really is something for everyone.

If you're not even remotely interested in any form of organized religion, that's totally fine, too. You should still seek out a time, place, or outlet for your own spiritual practice—whether it's a secular meditation or yoga class or a mindful hike in nature. The benefits to your brain are too great to ignore.

## THE SCIENCE OF SPIRITUALITY

When you look at the effects of prayer and meditation on the brain in scans, you can see why spiritual practice is so vital to us. We have the most evolved brains on the planet, and we have a responsibility to take special care of those brains. Most animals don't live as long as humans, nor do they get Alzheimer's disease or have spiritual crises. For better or worse, our brains set us apart.

It's been said that if the soul lived in a part of the brain, it would be in the prefrontal cortex, the part of our brains that most separates us from animals. The prefrontal cortex is one of the most uniquely "human" parts of the brain, associated with connection to others and long-term planning (in opposition to other, more primitive parts of the brain concerned with reward and short-term pleasure). And, remarkably enough, the prefrontal cortex can be exercised and even physically thickened through spiritual practice.

When the prefrontal cortex is active, it's associated with good mood. When it's not, it's associated with depression, anxiety, and addiction. Spiritual practice also positively affects other parts of the brain, like increasing activity in the anterior cingulate, which helps a person to feel more compassionate.

Both prayer and meditation can also *decrease* activity in the parietal lobe, a change that breaks down the boundaries people feel between themselves, the universe, nature, and God—talk about a stress reliever! This physiological mechanism also explains the sense of oneness that advanced prayer, meditation, and music trigger in people, and why some cultures have used psychedelics to achieve spiritual states. But it isn't necessary to take peyote or magic mushrooms: this state can be achieved just by sitting quietly in a room or on a beach and feeling a state of connectedness to all people.

Different faith traditions have a great deal in common—music, prayer, and meditation, an emphasis on morality, compassion, and love—and we could all benefit from focusing on these similarities instead of the differences. From a scientific point of view, Christians, Jews, Muslims, Buddhists, and even agnostics who meditate or pray all attain similar neurological states. These states are associated with compassion and connection, so there are also some common universal goals. A study of practices from different faith traditions—the rosary prayer and yoga mantras—shows *both* have positive psychological and even physiological benefits.[6] And brain scans conducted of nuns and Buddhists showed similar neurological changes as well.[7]

Whatever their religious traditions, devout people exercise the most evolved part of the brain, continuing to distance the human brain from the animal brain by gaining access to feelings of peace, compassion, and connection. We need all of these experiences to thrive, and too many of us aren't getting them.

## ACTION PLAN

Here are a few things you can do to get into the spiritual work:

**Explore Different Spiritual Paths:** Buy books about spiritual traditions that interest you. Attend some local services. Even if your first few visits aren't the perfect fit, look for the one or two lessons that could enhance your life. Begin a journey to embrace the beliefs that work best for you.

**Meditate More:** Even if you don't consider yourself to be a religious person, you can think and feel better by engaging in a spiritual practice in a secular way. Much of the research on meditation has focused on long-term meditators like monks and nuns who meditate for hours a day for decades. But here's the great news: You don't have to move to an ashram or devote your life to spiritual enlightenment to reap big benefits. Many begin to become apparent with only *12 minutes of practice a day!* And these changes surface in just weeks, not decades.

When acclaimed neuroscientist Dr. Andrew Newberg studied subjects with memory loss after they engaged in 12-minute daily meditations, brain scans showed that they had increased activity in the prefrontal cortex as well as increased blood flow to the brain. And while the meditation had no religious meaning attached to it for the subjects, their brains showed decreased activity in the parietal lobe, which results in a feeling of being at one with the universe, nature, or God—not bad for a 12-minute daily commitment! Subjects' memories also improved by an average of 10 to 20 percent, with some showing an improvement near 50 percent.[8]

Meditation and other mindfulness-based practices can ameliorate a huge range of both physical and mental illnesses: symptoms related to ADHD, addiction, depression, anxiety, cancer, heart disease, HIV, and insomnia. So before popping a stimulant like Adderall or Ritalin to treat ADHD, first enroll in a mindfulness meditation class, which research has shown to be very effective.[9] Or try the quick and easy techniques I introduce in the 7-Day Spirit Revolution beginning on page 219. Some of these meditations are adapted from Dr. Jon

Kabat-Zinn's Mindfulness-Based Stress Reduction (MBSR) program, which was later adapted into an effective treatment for depression: Mindfulness-Based Cognitive Therapy (MBCT).

**Explore the Great Outdoors:** Another way to cultivate a feeling of oneness with the universe is to spend more time in nature. As we trade walks in the forest for multitasking in front of the TV, computer, and cell phone, we fray our attention spans and become more prone to insomnia, anxiety, and other neurological ailments. Consider the fact that children spend only 15 to 25 minutes per day in outdoor play and sports and over 7½ hours per day engaged with media like TV, phones, and computers. It's no coincidence that kids in homes without computers spend more time outdoors.[10]

As we free ourselves from the dings and whistles that distract us, we can better appreciate the beauty, serenity, and stillness of nature—and our attention spans might improve as a result. One study found that merely looking at *slides* of nature photos improved attention in subjects.[11] If photos work that well, imagine what an encounter with actual nature might do!

And just as we *think* we're getting more done by multitasking but are actually wasting time, we're also *preventing* ourselves from our optimum performance by spending our lunch hour working in our cubicles. One study showed that after immersion in nature (which included disconnecting from technology), subjects improved 50 percent on a creative problem-solving task.[12]

You might be surprised by how much your whole life and outlook will change when you put down your phone and instead tune in to the world around you.

By now, you're probably excited to see just how easy it can be to take all of this information and apply it to your own life. Before I show you how to do that, I'd like to address two specific times people tend to notice dramatic changes in their brains: during pregnancy and old age. If you don't need to learn about mommy brain and senior moments, feel free to turn to page 171 to get started.

# PART V

# SPECIAL CARE FOR SPECIAL CASES

CHAPTER 14

# MOMMY BRAIN

Larissa was a senior partner at a prestigious law firm. She had worked hard to achieve so much by her mid-40s, but her world had been turned upside down with the birth of her new baby—which she had on her own, through in vitro fertilization. While Larissa made a good living and was able to hire both a housekeeper and a nanny to help her, she frequently felt overwhelmed by the combined demands of work and home.

When Larissa first came to see me, soon after she'd gone back to work and left her four-month-old with the nanny, she was close to tears. "Logically, I know I have everything I have ever wanted—the baby, the job, the financial independence . . . So why don't I *feel* more joy?" she asked me.

"And I forget *everything*, which is no big surprise considering how exhausted I am all the time. But is it ever going to get better? Am I going to feel this stressed out forever? I'm just going, going, going every minute, and most of the time, I feel like my brain isn't even functioning. The other day I came this close to making a major error that could have cost my client hundreds of thousands of dollars, and last week, I went to the grocery store for diapers and left without buying them." She shook her head as the tears began to stream down her face.

"Half the time I feel like I'm running at top speed," she said, "and the other half, I feel like I'm sleepwalking—it's like my brain has turned into Swiss cheese. When I'm working, I feel guilty that I'm not spending time with my son. But when I'm with my son, I can't help but think about all the things I need to be doing for work. Honestly, most of the time I just feel numb. I thought a baby would make my life complete—instead I feel totally lost."

She dried her eyes with a tissue and took a deep breath. "I never used to be like this!" she said, trying to compose herself. "What is happening to me?"

## DEALING WITH YOUR NEW PRIORITIES

Larissa is experiencing all the classic symptoms of mommy brain. She's a new mom who hasn't slept since God knows when. One minute she's ecstatic; the next minute she's depressed. She feels scatterbrained and worries that her memory just isn't as sharp as it used to be.

First things first: Larissa is not alone—and if you've experienced any of her symptoms, neither are you. In one study, over 80 percent of pregnant women reported impaired memory during pregnancy, which tests confirmed.[1] Research has shown verbal learning becomes more difficult as processing speed slows down.[2]

But motherhood doesn't damage the brain; it just rearranges priorities a bit. The phenomenon known as "mommy brain" is actually improving some areas of the brain while putting others on the back burner for a while. From an evolutionary point of view, a new mother has become the primary caretaker of a preverbal being who needs protection and bonding.

In a way, the mommy brain deficits in cognitive skills and verbal memory make sense. A newborn is at a crucial time of development, both physically and psychologically. The mother-child attachment creates a deep bond that makes the mother attuned to the child's every emotion and desire, to the unique sound of his cry and even his particular smell. She also becomes more aware of dangerous situations that might threaten him. As a consequence, a new mother's brain might shift to accommodate these new sensations. Cognitive skills and verbal memory just aren't as vital as bonding with and protecting a preverbal infant.

Brain scans of new mothers showed growth in the areas of the brain related to parent-child interaction, planning, parenting behavior, and warmth in the prefrontal cortex and amygdala. Researchers also had mothers select words from a list that described their babies. The most exuberant mothers actually showed the most growth.[3]

So savor this special time, which will be gone in a flash—even if it feels like it's dragging on forever. I've put together a few concrete strategies to help you enjoy your first months as a parent—without worrying too much about your brain. You'll get your old self back before you know it, and your life will be emotionally richer than ever before.

## ACTION PLAN

**Surrender to the Joys of Being a New Parent**. Playing peek-a-boo may not seem as stimulating as a big class-action lawsuit, but in reality it's more important. Cultivating a sense of gratitude will help you discover the many joys of parenthood while you form a bond with the most precious creature in your life. You'll also be nurturing your brain in the areas that prevent depression and anxiety.

**Eat an Anti-inflammatory Diet**. The natural inflammatory response that occurs at the end of a woman's pregnancy is the body's way of preventing infection after pregnancy. That means that new moms are subject to high levels of inflammation in addition to the roller coaster of hormones, both of which can contribute to depression. Not to worry: in the 7-Day Mood Revolution, you'll be swapping pro-inflammatory foods for anti-inflammatory ones.

**Increase Your Intake of the Omega-3s Found Primarily in Seafood: EPA and Especially DHA.** DHA, which is related to cognition, is essential to a developing infant's brain; that's why a pregnant woman's body passes on so much DHA to the fetus. It's unfortunate that so many pregnant women have eliminated all seafood from their diets when they should really be eating *more* seafood, cutting out only those fish like tuna and swordfish that have high toxin levels. One study showed the women who ate the least seafood during pregnancy had children who were more likely to have lower verbal IQ scores and poor social skills and motor skills.[4]

And it's not just your developing child who needs these omega-3s. You need them, too! If motherhood has depleted your reserves of omega-3s, your cognitive performance and mood might suffer. So make a concerted effort to get enough omega-3s from the clean fish recommended on pages 46 to 47. One study found greater seafood consumption and higher DHA levels in mothers' milk predicted lower rates of postpartum depression.[5] (Vegetarians can supplement with an algae-based DHA and the vegetarian omega-3 superfoods on page 182.)

Eating clean seafood also gives you the omega-3 EPA that is associated with preventing depression and decreasing anxiety—critical for new moms. You can't stop your levels of estrogen from skyrocketing during your pregnancy and plummeting after you give birth, but getting enough omega-3s may safeguard you from some of the moodiness and anxiety associated with this tumultuous (but brief, I promise!) life phase.

> **EXPERT'S TIP:** If you're a woman experiencing true postpartum depression, you should talk to your doctor right away about additional treatment options. The postpartum period is the most vulnerable time in a woman's life to experience depression. You need to know that it's not about not loving your baby. It's biology. It's temporary. And it's treatable.

**Fight the Bad Food Cravings.** The stress and sleep deprivation that come with new motherhood will make you crave processed carbs, which as we know release a burst of soothing serotonin. But be warned that this short-term fix actually makes mommy brain worse, since blood-sugar spikes can mess with your memory and cognition. Instead, try building your diet around the healthier carbs that will give your brain what it needs, like fiber to keep you full and amino acids like tryptophan that support natural serotonin production without spiking it. Pairing these foods with healthy, high-protein omega-3 sources and lots of vegetables will keep you full and happy—and far more capable of managing the inevitable stresses that come with motherhood.

**Sharpen Your Cognitive Skills.** The strategies in the 7-Day Energy Revolution will address some of a new mom's memory problems with a combination of brain training, exercise, and other activities that promote neurogenesis. My plan will allow you to continue to be that on-point attorney *and* a great mom. There's one other simple strategy to employ: relying more on your electronic calendar or written to-do list.

**Become More Mindful.** The spiritual principles and meditation practices you'll experiment with in the 7-Day Spirit Revolution will help strengthen your prefrontal cortex, which is associated with a sense of peace, connectedness, and equanimity. And you'll need all the calm you can get in the years to come: a recent study found that parents experienced more daily stress than nonparents. But the news isn't all grim, because the same study found that parents also experience more daily *joy* than nonparents.[6] In fact, another survey of thousands of people—parents, nonparents, single, cohabitating, married—found that moms were happier with life than any other group.

Mindfulness exercises also help you put the brakes on the urge to curse or throw things during those extremely low moments inevitable in parenthood. A strengthened prefrontal cortex gives you the tranquility to get through even the toughest moments with your kids. These mindfulness principles are also vital to moms since so many moms are notorious multitaskers. Of course, moms sometimes need to multitask, but as we learned in Chapter 11 on digital distraction, multitasking doesn't actually save time. So whenever you can, try to employ the mindfulness practices I introduce in week 3 that will help you do one thing (and only one thing) at a time.

**Sleep When You Can.** The sleep principles in Chapter 10 are doubly important for new moms (while, of course, being harder to adhere to). Many of the memory deficits new moms experience are likely related to a lack of sleep. Who wouldn't feel scattered on four hours a night? Sleep at night whenever you can—even if it means turning in at 8 P.M.—and supplement with short afternoon naps. Now that you know how vital sleep is to mood and memory, you shouldn't feel guilty asking the in-laws to pick up an occasional nighttime shift. If you're co-parenting, alternate the nighttime shifts so that one of you is getting a good night's sleep every other night, as opposed to both of you getting a fair to poor night's sleep every night.

Another trick is to swap out the compact fluorescent bulbs, which have higher levels of circadian rhythm–disrupting blue light, in your room for incandescent bulbs on a dimmer or the Good Night light bulb, which will help you get back to sleep after your baby's nighttime wakeups.

**Step 8: Remember It's Only Temporary!** For all the tribulations and stresses of this time of life, this period will be over before you know it. And though you may feel scattered, you're also becoming a more connected, empathic parent. And by following the principles in my 21-day program, you can address many of the temporary deficits that you might be experiencing.

CHAPTER 15

# Senior Moments

Ward was a broad-shouldered, boisterous man in his early 70s who was visibly upset when he came into my office. A retired military man, Ward had a loud voice and a precise way of speaking. He was clearly anxious as he described several incidents in which he'd been "not up to par," as he put it: the other day when he couldn't remember the name of an old colleague; the evening when he forgot where he parked his car. And more and more often, he couldn't retrieve the right word on demand.

Even into his 60s, Ward had always felt as mentally sharp as the 30-somethings who worked with him. That began to change soon after he retired. He had been trying to do more crossword puzzles, but they didn't seem to help. A neurologist ran some tests and assured Ward that what he was experiencing was just normal, age-related cognitive decline and said there wasn't much he could do about it. What most worried Ward were the Alzheimer's disease stats the neurologist shared with him: one in eight for people 65 or older and over half of those over 85.

You see, Ward had lived his life as a "beat the odds" kind of guy. He was born in a trailer and had worked two different jobs in high school to help his family and to save for college—the first of his family ever to attend. He was not a guy who was going to take old age lying down.

"All four of my grandparents lived into their nineties, and all four of 'em were sharp as a tack! And here I am, seventy-two years old and failing," Ward said. "Help me out here, Doc."

I quickly assured Ward that, although he was getting older, he didn't have to lose his edge and surrender to "senior moments." In fact, brand-new research suggests memory loss may be reversible. The right diet and exercise could make a world of difference in clearing away his brain fog and promoting neurogenesis, the brain's ability to grow and change when presented with new challenges.

A simple memory game called the n-back, the addition of an inexpensive spice into his daily diet, and some new skills might provide Ward with the chance for his brain to stretch, grow, and sharpen.

## WHAT MILD COGNITIVE IMPAIRMENT MEANS— AND WHAT YOU CAN DO ABOUT IT

Beginning in the late 1990s, the term *mild cognitive impairment* kept popping up in medical journals and magazine articles. And in 2013, *DSM-5, The Diagnostic and Statistical Manual of Mental Disorders* from the American Psychiatric Association, added *mild neurocognitive disorder* to its list of official diagnoses.

All sorts of related terms—*age-associated memory impairment, subjective cognitive impairment,* or, my personal favorite, *"senior moments"*—refer to that gray area between normal functioning and dementia or Alzheimer's disease. These recommendations don't just apply to the 65-and-over set, however. The time to take care of your brain starts much earlier. Research shows your brain starts to noticeably slow down by your 40s, particularly if you do nothing to combat it. One study that tested over 7,000 people over the course of a decade found that *all* cognitive skills tested except vocabulary declined.[1] If you work on sharpening your cognitive skills earlier in life, you will reap the benefits decades later.[2] As baby boomers get older and our life spans lengthen (and as we eat more processed carbs, move less, and gain weight), mild cognitive impairment has seemed to take on epidemic proportions.

Up to 17 percent of people over 65 may have some form of mild cognitive impairment, but what exactly *is* it?[3] Signs of mild cognitive impairment include difficulty in these areas:

- Remembering names
- Finding the correct word
- Remembering where objects are located
- Concentrating

Many of these symptoms might not seem all that serious at first glance, so if you're of a certain age and have had any of these problems, you might be thinking, *Well, that doesn't sound so bad. And even if it is bad, it's not as if I can do anything about it.*

Wrong on both counts. Between 6 to 15 percent of patients who meet criteria for mild cognitive impairment will receive a diagnosis of dementia every year. After ten years, up to 80 percent of them will have or—if they've passed away—have had Alzheimer's.

And, as we know, Alzheimer's disease is challenging to treat, financially disastrous, and, of course, emotionally devastating. It's already the sixth leading cause of death in the U.S. and in 2013, a new report from the journal *Neurology* warned that by 2050, the number of Americans with Alzheimer's disease will triple from the 5 million currently to almost 14 million.

That said, if you're diagnosed with mild cognitive impairment, you are by no means doomed to an eventual Alzheimer's diagnosis. On the contrary, take it as all the more reason to go on the offensive. There are *so many* things you can do to prevent and even reverse age-related types of cognitive decline. If your memory is going, you can fight to get it back.

One part of the brain involved in learning and memory, the hippocampus, is especially vulnerable to aging, and it produces less and less of the key protein RbAp48. In one study, inhibiting this protein in young mice's brains made them forgetful in mazes. But when scientists *increased* this protein in old mice, their memories and cognitive performance were similar to those of young mice.[4] Now that's encouraging!

While injecting this protein directly into our brains isn't an option for now, we certainly can employ neurogenesis-boosting strategies that keep the hippocampus fit, and potentially even reverse decline that's already occurring.

The young-and-old-mice study also provided evidence that age-related memory loss and Alzheimer's disease are two distinct conditions. Normal age-related decline targets the hippocampus, whereas Alzheimer's disease takes a different route, initially targeting a region of the brain called the entorhinal cortex.

And though "senior moments" and Alzheimer's are distinct conditions, you can slow down or even prevent both. Very few cases of Alzheimer's—only about 10 percent—are inherited.

## TAKING CHARGE OF YOUR AGING BRAIN

We will be targeting two primary brain structures in this program, both of which are involved in learning as well as short- and long-term memory: the hippocampus and the prefrontal cortex. When we strengthen these two areas, we can go a long way toward fighting senior moments.

The hippocampus is the principal site of neurogenesis in the brain, which means we can actually grow new brain cells with the strategies we will use in the 7-Day Energy Revolution. We can also physically increase the thickness of the prefrontal cortex through meditation, part of the 7-Day Spirit Revolution. (This is especially important as the prefrontal cortex begins to shrink in middle adulthood while simultaneously losing dopamine.)

## ACTION PLAN

**Never Stop Learning:** The most reliable way to keep your brain sharp is to make learning a lifelong pursuit. Learn when you're young, and once you're done with school and in your chosen career, keep on learning. Learning is especially important as you get older, especially after retirement.

Learning is one of the best tools to protect the brain from cognitive decline and senior moments. It's why people with higher levels of education have fewer senior moments, and why people who speak only one language show symptoms of dementia four years before bilinguals.[5]

Learning also increases your cognitive reserve—it builds neurons and connections in your brain. The more of these you have, the more you can spare. It's not just about preventing Alzheimer's-causing plaques from building up by using strategies like sleeping eight hours a night. People who have built their cognitive reserves through learning can continue to function well even *after* the plaques have started to develop. And whatever our level of education or genetics, we all have the capability to grow more neurons and connections.

So as soon as you put down this book, head over to the Learning Annex, or your local library. Download a lecture online. Take up astronomy, or gardening, or any other subject that strikes your fancy.

**Have Fun:** In addition to learning, staying engaged in leisure activities helps you stimulate your brain. One famous study looked at almost 500 elderly people to examine the relationship between leisure activities and cognitive decline. Reading, playing board games and musical instruments, and dancing all reduced subjects' risk of cognitive decline.[6] Another study found traveling, gardening, and knitting also have protective effects.[7] Yet another identified activities like reading and playing board games as protective against senior moments. But notably, there was one activity that *significantly increased* the risk of cognitive decline: watching TV. While reading reduced the risk of cognitive impairment by about 5 percent, watching TV *increased* the risk by 20 percent![8] So if you want to curtail senior moments, start by watching less TV and doing more gardening, card playing, or traveling.

**Get Moving:** Exercise is another fun activity that can protect your brain against cognitive decline. Aerobic activity has been shown to promote neurogenesis in the hippocampus.[9] Just the simple act of walking every day might cut the risk of dementia in elderly people in half.[10]

Another study found aerobic exercise in older adults led to increases in brain volume in areas associated with cognition.[11] And still another study found that the more people walked, the larger their brain volume (which was associated with a lower risk of mild cognitive impairment).[12]

Exercise is also important because it helps reduce belly fat, and carrying excess belly weight can spell bad news for the brain. In one study, people with the most belly fat were three times more likely to develop dementia than those with the least. Even those subjects who did not have excess belly fat but were overweight had an 80 percent increased risk of developing dementia.[13]

Exercise is also an extremely effective natural antidepressant, which becomes doubly important as people get older, since prescription antidepressants can impair cognition.[14] And since older people are more likely to be on other medications—many of which are vital to their health—they should be all the more proactive about employing natural strategies to decrease the total number of pills they take for all conditions.

**Do the N-Back Task:** The other miracle memory treatment is something you will start doing during the 7-Day Energy Revolution for 12 minutes a day. It's called the n-back task (see page 188 for instructions). If you've ever played the childhood game *Concentration,* you've used a version of this. And most brain training systems and apps like Lumosity and BrainHQ use a version of this as well. But you don't need a subscription. You can just turn to the Appendix A on page 237 and start playing it now.

Unlike strategies that target crystallized intelligence, the knowledge and skills you acquire through life experience (such as expanding your vocabulary through crossword puzzles), the n-back targets your working memory, which tends to decline as you get older.

Crystallized intelligence, on the other hand, increases throughout most of the life span. You learn more facts, and you become better at *Trivial Pursuit.* But working memory is important because it allows you to hold information for a short amount of time while also being able to manipulate that information if necessary. Many of life's more complex tasks require you to tap into this type of memory.

But what's truly remarkable about the n-back task is that, for all its simplicity, it's been shown to actually improve *fluid* intelligence, which is vital for learning and was once thought of as fairly unchangeable. Because fluid intelligence generally declines after young adulthood, it's one of the most important kinds of intelligence to improve if you want to prevent senior moments.

It doesn't take a huge commitment to see the gains, either. You can improve your memory by doing the n-back task for just 25 minutes a day or even less in just a week, with even more gains after a few weeks.[15] The n-back task even helped 80-year-olds improve their memories.[16]

**Eat Smart:** We've discussed overhauling your diet throughout the book, and luckily, all of the dietary changes we'll be making in the 7-Day Mood Revolution—decreasing blood-sugar spikes, shifting from omega-6 to omega-3 proteins and fats, moving from soybean to olive oil, and eating lots of vegetables and legumes high in B vitamins, including folate—will work wonders to prevent senior moments and other forms of cognitive decline.

The Brain Fog Fix Program is, generally speaking, an amped-up version of the Mediterranean diet, which has been associated with a lower risk of mild cognitive impairment. For people who already have mild cognitive impairment, this diet will help prevent a transition from mild cognitive impairment to Alzheimer's disease.[17] We will be building our diets around Mediterranean basics like fish and olive oil as well as dramatically cutting back on processed carbs, choosing organic and pasture-raised meats and dairy, and eating a record-breaking seven servings of vegetables and fruits every day.

We will focus on a few specific foods that are particularly good for preventing senior moments, namely berries, turmeric, and fish.

- **Berries:** Berries are truly a miracle food for your brain—high in flavonoids as well as fiber, which manages blood-sugar spikes—not to mention being delicious. Eating berries regularly has been shown to slow the progression of cognitive decline by up to 2½ years, according to one study.[18] Blueberries in particular might even help people overcome genetic predispositions for Alzheimer's disease.[19] Berries may have the power to reverse age-related decline according to one study.[20]

  So tomorrow at breakfast, ditch the orange juice and toast and reach for the slow-burning carbs in blueberries and raspberries. Mix in them in protein shakes with organic milk or unsweetened almond milk, or eat them with stevia and plain Greek yogurt.

- **Fish:** We've already seen how the omega-3s in fish, DHA and EPA, can improve the functioning of our brain, and this becomes particularly important as we age. One recent study with adults aged 50 to 75 found that verbal fluency, visual tasks, and reading ability all improved with a fish oil supplement. The fish oil even helped improve the structure of the brain itself.[21] Another study showed that an omega-3 supplement could improve working memory.[22] And fish isn't just prevention but also *treatment.* In a study of subjects who were already experiencing senior moments, the ones taking a DHA supplement showed improved verbal fluency after six months.[23] The omega-3 superfoods you will be eating beginning with the 7-Day Mood Revolution will help ensure that you're getting enough EPA and DHA.

- **Turmeric:** And then there's the most miraculous brain-restoring ingredient of all, which we discussed earlier: turmeric. The effects of this miracle spice are quite evident in rural India, where fewer than 1 percent of seniors aged 65 and over have Alzheimer's disease, compared to about 13 percent in the United States. The reason for this discrepancy is shockingly simple and incredibly inexpensive: it's because Indians eat a lot of turmeric, a spice used in curry that contains curcumin, which has major anti-inflammatory and antioxidant properties.

Turmeric can also increase brain-derived neurotrophic factor, which enhances neurogenesis in the brain while fighting Alzheimer's disease–causing plaques. One study showed that turmeric helps the body clear brain-fogging plaques from the brain.[24] Another found evidence of neurogenesis and enhanced cognition in older rats in as little as 12 weeks.[25] And in addition to making you *think* better, turmeric will make you *feel* better, too, possibly increasing serotonin in the brain.[26]

Try to get a little of this magical spice regularly, not just once a month when you wind up at an Indian restaurant, for low doses of turmeric over a long period of time are more effective than very occasional high doses in fighting Alzheimer's disease–causing plaques.[27] And remember: try to eat it with black pepper as the Indians do in curry. That makes it even more powerful because this combo makes the turmeric bioavailable.

- **Other Great Spices:** Saffron, another common ingredient in curry, can also inhibit Alzheimer's disease–causing plaques.[28] Try adding dashes of saffron to organic chicken. Rosemary is another herb that works wonders. The carnosic acid in rosemary may also reduce your risk of Alzheimer's disease, while the scent alone can improve memory.[29] Spanish sage has been shown to improve word recall, a common "senior moment" complaint.[30] The moral of the story here: lots of herbs and spices. So put down the salt and flavor your food with any other herb or spice. Your brain and your taste buds will both thank you.

# PART VI:

# THE
# BRAIN FOG
# FIX
# PROGRAM

CHAPTER 16

# Program Overview

Now for the fun part—actually taking charge of your life and re-forming your brain-fogging habits over the next 21 days! The program is broken up into three weeks, with a special focus during each. In the first week, you'll be cleaning up your diet and supercharging your mood by changing the way you think. In the second week, you'll be revving up your energy levels and increasing your ability to focus. In the final week, you will begin searching for the spiritual connection that's missing from so many modern lives.

## Your Three-Week Program

### WEEK 1: THE 7-DAY MOOD REVOLUTION

Change your diet to go from unbalanced and listless to revitalized and energetic. Use cognitive strategies to help change the way you think, focusing on one of the seven pitfall thought patterns each day.

### WEEK 2: THE 7-DAY ENERGY REVOLUTION

Use sleep, circadian rhythms, exercise, and *neurogenesis* to go from foggy and scattered to alert and sharp. (*Neurogenesis* is the ability of your brain to grow and change when it is stimulated and learning new things.) Use behavioral strategies to help change what you do.

### WEEK 3: THE 7-DAY SPIRIT REVOLUTION

Connect to something larger than yourself to recommit your life's purpose and rediscover your joy in life.

In the following pages, I'll go through in depth what each week will entail, and then in the next chapter, I'll take you by the hand and walk you through each of the 21 days. We'll make this as painless and brain clearing, mood boosting, and energy renewing as possible.

Keep in mind that the strategies you will learn are designed to help you integrate the healthy practices in this program for the rest of your life. While I'll ask you to stick strictly to what I've outlined for each week, after that I ask you to continue the work following my 80/20 rule—hopefully for the rest of your life, but at least for the three weeks of the program. So, for example, in week 1, you will eat an omega-3 superfood and seven vegetables and fruits every single day while cutting out sugar and flour entirely. After week 1, I hope that you will eat an omega-3 superfood, seven vegetables and fruits, and very little flour or sugar every day *for the rest of your life!* The same goes for everything you add through this program—from exercise to meditation. This will ensure that you continue to think and feel better and better!

So let's jump in now to the explanation of what you'll be doing in these three stages of the program.

## WEEK 1: THE 7-DAY MOOD REVOLUTION

During the first week, we're going to take you from unbalanced to revitalized by focusing on two critical areas:

**Diet:** We will be removing the problematic foods that cause brain-fogging blood-sugar spikes and inflammation. And we'll be adding foods that heal, nourish, and support your brain.

**Cognition:** Each day, you'll begin to transform your thoughts by noticing one of my seven pitfall thought patterns each day. Just by becoming aware of these pitfall thought patterns, you'll come to realize that by changing the way you *think*, you can also begin to change the way you *feel*, which has a remarkable power to change how you act and the choices you make.

Okay, let's take on the diet first. Some of these changes might seem a little intimidating at first, but don't worry—once you've completed this week, you can get a little less intense. After one week of intense work, just live by the 80/20 rule we discussed in Chapter 3 for at least the rest of the program (and preferably your whole life!). In the meantime, I must warn you that it may get worse before it gets better, so don't start the program on a busy Monday morning when work is crazy. It'll be far more effective if you start on a quiet weekend when you can really devote yourself to making these changes. Before you know it, you'll be enjoying an enduring energy boost from the infusion of B vitamins and other nutrients that far too many of us are neglecting.

## DIET OVERHAUL

To overhaul our diets, we're going to address six things; the first four are what we're going to cut out of our diets, and the last two are all about adding:

1. Sugar and artificial sweeteners

2. Flour and processed snacks

3. Pro-inflammatory omega-6s

4. Caffeine, alcohol, and any other substances that put you on a hormonal roller coaster

5. Omega-3 superfoods

6. Fruits and vegetables

Our very first step is to cut out the blood sugar–spiking foods (discussed in detail in Chapter 3, page 25) that can lead to inflammation, brain fog, and depression. This might actually be the very hardest step in the whole process for many of us, since the average American eats way too many of these foods.

As I walk you through what we will be cutting out, I'll also offer a range of suggestions for foods that you could start trying out as possible replacements. And then we get to the fun part—adding food in.

### Say Good-Bye to Sugar and Artificial Sweeteners

Sugar is a major culprit in the up-and-down mood roller coaster many of us experience. There is a strong link between high-sugar diets and neurodegenerative conditions like dementia and even Alzheimer's.

**Eliminate:**

- All sugar
- High-fructose corn syrup, corn syrup, corn syrup solids
- Any other kinds of syrup: carob syrup, golden syrup, malt syrup, maple syrup
- Most words ending in "ose," such as: dextrose, fructose, galactose, glucose, maltose, sucrose
- Dextrin or maltodextrin

- Agave

- Honey

- Fruit juice or "sweetened with fruit juice"

- Artificial sweeteners: sucralose (Splenda), aspartame (Nutrasweet), saccharin (Sweet'N Low), acesulfame potassium (Acesulfame K, Ace K, Sunett, Sweet One, E950)

**Replace With:** You are going to learn to appreciate the natural sweetness of fruits, but if you still need some sweetener in your life, I consider stevia (Rebiana, Truvia, Pure Via) an acceptable substitute. You can get it in packets or in zero-calorie beverages like Vitaminwater Zero.

**Sweet Substitutions:** You don't have to give up dessert to feed your brain! Once you give up overly sweetened processed carbs, you will be utterly amazed by the natural sweetness of foods.

- Swap fruit-flavored yogurt for plain Greek yogurt.

- For dessert, try organic, plain Greek yogurt with organic blueberries and stevia.

- A delicious smoothie with 80 percent vegetables and 20 percent fruit. (See "A Blender, a Bottle, and a Buck" on page 247 for some great suggestions.)

- I also love Quest Protein Bars, which are made from whey protein (whereas most protein bars are made from cheap, nonorganic soy protein isolate). While some of the flavors use artificial sweeteners, many don't. Look for the flavors that say "no artificial sweeteners" on the front. I particularly like the Quest Chocolate Peanut Butter bar. Twenty seconds in the microwave and you have my go-to dessert.

**Better Beverages:** Since beverages are often a *huge* source of sugar in the diet, you can bring down your glycemic load a great deal simply by making smoothies and juices with an 80/20 ratio of veggies to fruit. (And since fresh lemons and limes contain just about one gram of sugar, you can count them as vegetables, too! They do wonders for adding a citrus taste to bitter vegetables.)

You may soon find that you prefer the taste of vegetables blended with fruit to those overly sweetened "smoothies" they sell at mall food courts, or even the bottled "green" ones that are marketed as vegetable juice but are made mostly of cheap, blood sugar–spiking fruits or apple juice. The drink will come out especially delicious if you blend the whole fruit (which keeps the skin and the fiber).

> **RECIPE:** My favorite: ¼ cup romaine, ¼ cup kale, ¼ cup spinach, ¼ cup broccoli, ¼ cucumber, a squeeze of lemon, a 1-inch piece of ginger, ½ pear with the skin on, a few pieces of cut mango, and 2 cups water. To make these as convenient as a bag of chips, I make 3 to 4 at a time and use wide-mouth Ball jars with lids to store in the fridge. Toss in your bag and go!

## Ditch the Flour and Processed Snacks

Flour (even those virtuous-looking whole-wheat varieties) has a through-the-roof glycemic index, meaning it raises your blood-sugar levels—the state we are trying to avoid. For the duration of the Mood Revolution, we will be cutting out all foods that contain flour as well as several other high-GI foods like potatoes and white rice.

**Eliminate:**

- All flour
- All bread containing flour
- Pasta

- Tortillas
- Chips
- Potatoes
- White rice

**Replace With:** You are going to learn to love these alternative carbohydrate sources. You can have up to two cups a day of these amazing foods:

- Brown rice
- Quinoa
- Barley
- Oatmeal
- Bulgur wheat
- Millet
- Couscous
- Spelt
- Flourless and sprouted grain bread

**Bread Alternatives:** I love flourless sprouted bread and English muffins, which provide energy-boosting carbs while cutting the glycemic index in half. My favorite is Ezekiel Food for Life 4:9, which you can get in just about any supermarket. These breads also provide brain-healthy amino acids and more protein than other types of bread. I like to toast my flourless bread, as it improves the texture.

**Some Other Suggestions:**

- At home, try a pizza made with portobello mushrooms instead of dough.
- Instead of chips, eat nuts (find plain ones that aren't cooked in oil).

- Make your own fried rice at home, with only ½ cup brown rice per serving (a big difference from restaurant fried rice, which is almost all rice). Make the bulk of your home-cooked dish with organic egg or meats, onions, chopped broccoli, red pepper, and diced carrots. Use just a tablespoon or two of olive oil to sauté, and finish with ginger, soy sauce, turmeric, and black pepper.

- Keep large leaves of romaine to use in place of bread for sandwiches.

**Healthier Sides and Snacks:** We also get a lot of blood sugar–spiking carbs from the snack foods we munch on all day and night. Luckily, it is incredibly easy to swap out these foods with healthier alternatives. Your brain (and your waistline) will thank you!

- Instead of nachos, try celery with salsa.

- Instead of pita chips, try cut red peppers, baby carrots, and cherry tomatoes with your hummus.

- Instead of crackers, try organic olive oil popcorn from Trader Joe's, or make your own brain-healthy microwave popcorn. See page 97 for a quick how-to.

- Instead of wheat toast with peanut butter, try apples or celery with almond butter.

- Instead of mashed potatoes, try making cauliflower mashed "potatoes" or mashed garbanzo beans.

**Pasta Alternatives:** Trust me, I of all people know how hard it is to live without pasta—since childhood, my biggest pitfall food has been bright-orange-powder macaroni and cheese straight out of the box. After week 1, feel free to indulge occasionally—remember 80/20. Here are some pretty simple, brain-benefiting swaps.

- Substitute shirataki noodles for pasta. These plant-based noodles have almost no carbohydrates. While once found only at health food and Asian stores, they're now available at pretty much any grocery store.

- Instead of pasta salad, make a black bean and corn salad.

## Ditch Foods That Are High in Pro-Inflammatory Omega-6s

Correcting the omega-3 to omega-6 ratio in our diets—which at the moment is completely out of whack—is one of the most important steps we can take to fight inflammation, brain fog, and depression. One of the major sources of omega-6s are conventionally raised animal products, so we will be getting rid of those right away. Remember, organic animal products might cost more up front, but you will be saving big in long-term health outcomes.

### Eliminate:

- Conventionally raised, nonorganic, or grain-fed meat, dairy, and eggs
- Fried foods
- All oils except for the four options listed below

### Replace With:

- Meat, dairy, and eggs labeled with one of the following words: organic, grass-fed, pastured, free-roaming, or free-range
- Extra virgin olive oil, olive oil, canola oil, flaxseed oil

**Oils, Dressings, and Sauces: A Few Condiment-Shopping Tips:** My favorite marinara sauces are the $3 per bottle premium line at Trader Joe's, which are extremely affordable and use *only* olive oil. (The second best choices are blends of olive and canola.)

Because some premium bottled salad dressings can cost more than $5, I recommend making your own salad dressings with extra virgin olive oil and vinegar. They'll save you money—and they taste much better, too. And since restaurant vinaigrettes are sometimes made with soybean oil, your safest bet is to ask for vinegar and olive oil.

Knowing where to shop helps, too. Start doing some of your grocery shopping online. I buy my reduced-fat Kraft olive oil mayonnaise on Amazon and get six easy-out squeeze bottles for $15. That's just a few bucks a bottle! (It's not perfect, as it does contain some soybean oil, so avoid this for week 1 of the program; when you read the ingredient label, however, you'll find olive oil is listed first, which means it contains more olive than soybean oil. Hellman's brand, which claims that it's "made with olive oil" on the front of the bottle, actually lists soybean oil first, which in my opinion is very misleading to the consumer. Avoid this one.) If you have the means, mayonnaise with *all* olive oil is absolutely delicious and compatible with the week 1 program, but these often run in the $10 per bottle range.

### Reduce Roller-Coaster Substances

Don't worry: we won't be eliminating these substances altogether. But we will attempt to reduce their impact on our circadian rhythms in anticipation of the next week. So for this week, you will limit yourself to natural unsweetened coffee (no energy drinks!) and moderate amounts of alcohol.

- A maximum of 200 mg caffeine per day (about two small cups of coffee)

**EXPERT'S TIP:** If you're used to sipping coffee all day long, try switching to green tea in the first few weeks of the program. You can have four to six cups a day without going over the 200 mg limit. Or, order half-caff coffee so you can have up to four small cups a day.

- A maximum of one serving of alcohol per day (preferably red wine). One serving is one glass of wine, one 8-ounce beer, or 1.5 ounces of liquor.

- No recreational drugs or smoking. (Note: This is not a program to treat drug or alcohol addiction.)

- If you are taking excess prescription medications, such as sleeping pills or benzodiazepines, you may wish to talk to your prescriber about tapering off or adjusting your dose after you have completed the 21-day program. The changes in diet, exercise, sleep hygiene, and lifestyle can often make this an ideal time to cut back on overmedication as your mood and energy improve.

## Add At Least One *Omega-3 Superfood* Per Day

Okay, now that I've told you everything you *can't* have, let's get into the good stuff that you should be adding to your diet, namely fish, fish, and more fish. During this first week, you are going to eat a serving of brain-nourishing omega-3 superfood *every single day*. Favor seafood-based superfoods since they give your brain the most concentrated doses of the two types of omega-3s, DHA and EPA. Ideally, you will have at least one serving of one of these fish per day:

- Albacore tuna, troll or pole caught, fresh or canned, U.S. or British Columbia
- Arctic char, farmed
- Barramundi, farmed, U.S.
- Black cod
- Dungeness crab, wild, California, Oregon, or Washington
- Longfin squid, wild, Atlantic
- Mussels, farmed
- Oysters, farmed
- Pacific sardines, wild
- Rainbow trout, farmed

- Spot prawns, wild, British Columbia
- Salmon, coho, farmed, U.S.
- Salmon, wild, any origin
- Shrimp

The other omega-3 superfoods are the following vegetarian options. However, these contain high levels of ALA, which your body must convert to DHA and EPA in order for you to think and feel better, and it doesn't do this very efficiently, especially in men. Vegetarian sources of ALA include:

- Walnuts (¼ cup)
- Flaxseeds, ground (2 tablespoons) or oil (1 tablespoon)
- Chia seeds (2 tablespoons)

**Shopping Tips:** A lot of the healthiest fish, like wild salmon, can be expensive, but with a little creativity you can get your daily dose of wild salmon for just over $1. I stock my pantry with vacuum-packed pouches of Chicken of the Sea Premium Wild-Caught Pink Salmon, which tastes like chunk light tuna—your kids won't be able to tell the difference—but has far more brain benefits than traditional tuna, with 500 mg of DHA and EPA per serving. If you can't find these packs at grocery stores, you can usually get them at Target or on Amazon for just over $1 a (BPA-free) pouch. Mix the salmon with some olive-oil-based mayonnaise and lemon juice, toast in a toaster oven or under a broiler with a slice of organic cheese on sprouted bread, and you've got an easy, inexpensive, and brain-healthy salmon melt.

**EXPERT'S TIP**: When it comes to tuna, the "premium" whole white albacore actually has about three times *more* mercury than the very inexpensive chunk light tuna—but both still contain mercury and neither is a great source of omega-3s. You'll never regret making the switch to wild salmon!

I also love the frozen meal line Artisan Bistro, which has lots of sustainably caught wild salmon meals for about $5. Cheaper lines of frozen meals usually contain about two ounces less than Artisan Bistro meals. In addition to being lower in protein, they generally contain higher levels of cheap, blood sugar–spiking processed carbs.

## Eat at Least Seven Servings of Vegetables and Whole Fruit Per Day

The next thing you will add to your diet in week 1 is at least seven servings of vegetables and whole fruit per day. You now know just how incredibly beneficial this simple strategy can be for mood, energy, and cognition. Here are a few general guidelines that will help you to get the maximum benefit from these disease-fighting, brain-boosting powerhouses:

- Favor vegetables over fruits.

- Favor berries among all fruits.

- Favor organic over conventionally grown.

- Eat a variety of vegetables and fruits to ensure you're getting the different vitamins that serve as cofactors and different antioxidants that prevent inflammation.

- When eating fruit, ensure that it's eaten whole or blended. Don't juice it.

- My favorite way to get enough servings of vegetables and fruit each day is to blend them. See page 247 for my "A Blender, a Bottle, and a Buck," which features my favorite juices. You can put them in portable Ball jars, and they cost less than $1 a serving.

To get the most out of the produce you're eating, you should also drink at least *ten eight-ounce servings* of water each day.

Now that wasn't so hard, was it? The other part of week 1 is a series of cognitive exercises that will help reshape the way you look at the world—and yourself.

## COGNITION OVERHAUL

I honestly believe that the dietary overhaul is the hardest part of this whole program. Eating well plays a massive role in overhauling your mood. But it's by no means the only element.

And you may find that while you are making such radical changes to the way you eat, you fall prey to some unhelpful thought patterns, which I, as a cognitive behavioral therapist, specialize in identifying. To combat this possibility, on every day of this week you will focus on one of what I call the "7 pitfall thought patterns" and try to work through it in a positive way. Once you can focus on the types of thought patterns that make you feel bad, you can reframe your thoughts in a more helpful light. These practices will help get you through the hardest part of leaving behind the brain-fogging foods you love so much!

Each day, you will be watching out for one of the seven pitfall thought patterns that can leave you thinking and feeling badly:

- **Personalization**: Assuming that something is happening because of you. ("I didn't get that job because I'm not smart enough.")

- **Pervasiveness**: Allowing a problem in your life to invade all parts of your life. ("I have a headache—might as well call in sick to work today.")

- **Paralysis-analysis**: Getting stuck in your own thoughts. ("Why couldn't I remember where I put my keys last night? What does it mean? What will I do if this keeps happening?")

- **Pessimism**: Always believing the worst about everything. ("I felt foggy this morning—I must be getting dementia.")

- **Polarization:** Seeing everything as either/or, black/white, yes/no. ("My boss didn't respond well to my presentation—I might as well just quit.")
- **Psychic:** Feeling sure that you know what another person is thinking. ("I know she's never liked me anyway.")
- **Permanence:** Using the past or present to judge the future. ("I'm never going to get over this divorce.")

By choosing to pay special attention to each pitfall thought pattern, you'll notice how often it tends to show up in your life. This awareness is the first step. Through this process—and a related daily evaluation process—you'll learn which pitfall thought patterns are the ones you engage in the most and how to reduce the number of times you engage in them. In doing so, you'll remove the mental blocks that prevent you from reaching your full potential. Like all the strategies you'll use throughout the course of your 21-day program, continue to be conscious of all the seven pitfall thought patterns even when you're not paying special attention to just one.

## WEEK 2: THE 7-DAY ENERGY REVOLUTION

In the second week of the program, we're going to get you from exhausted to energized by focusing on:

1. **Sleep and circadian rhythms:** Adjust your brain's relationship to natural light to regulate your sleep rhythms and boost your energy.

2. **Exercise:** Give your body the exercise your brain needs to stay active and support neuron growth.

3. **Neurogenesis:** Keep learning new things to enhance your brain, because if you're not moving forward, you're sliding backward. You will also eat one neurogenesis superfood containing turmeric and black pepper every single day.

4. **Attention and reward:** Cutting back on social media and electronics will boost your ability to focus and concentrate while restoring your ability to experience joy in life.

## GET TO SLEEP!

Your new and improved diet has probably already altered your sleep habits for the better. Without constant blood-sugar spikes from processed carbohydrates and an excess of caffeine and alcohol to mess with your circadian rhythms, you are probably getting deeper rest as a matter of course. But there are a few more steps you can take to ensure even more restorative sleep every night.

The goal is to get about eight hours of restful sleep each night if at all possible, which might mean going to bed earlier than you're accustomed to doing. Get to bed by 11 P.M. and wake by 7 A.M., and keep your sleep and wake times constant throughout the week: these natural cycles are crucial for good health. Expose yourself to bright light soon after waking by opening all shades, turning on all lights, using a light box, or going outside immediately.

Promote good sleep hygiene for deep sleep using the following techniques:

- No television.

- No computer or tablet use after 7 P.M.

- Replace all fluorescent bulbs to which you are exposed after 7 P.M. with incandescent or LED bulbs with a dimmer to keep the light output as low as possible to prevent eye strain.

- Wear sunglasses after 7 P.M. when outside when there is any sunlight present.

- Allow your eyes to be exposed to sunlight in the morning and during the day. Go outside. Open blinds during the day, and turn your desk toward windows.

- If you live in a climate where you do not get ample sunlight year round, buy a full-spectrum or blue light box to use for 15 to 20 minutes first thing in the morning and again in the early afternoon. These are available for less than $50. (Do not use these if you have ever been diagnosed with bipolar disorder as they may trigger manic episodes.)

- If there is any light at all in your bedroom, either install blackout shades or use a sleep mask.

- Keep your room cool, around 68 degrees. Make sure that your feet are warm, though, wearing socks if you need to warm them.

- For night-shift workers, ensure that you mimic a natural circadian response by exposing yourself to bright light during your working hours and at least eight hours of complete darkness when you are sleeping. Also consider Definity Digital's light bulbs that I suggest on page 123.

## GET MOVING!

Get 44 minutes of aerobic exercise per day minimum to stimulate the *dentate gyrus* of your hippocampus, the area of the brain linked to memory, mood, and stress. When you stimulate your dentate gyrus, you help support *neurogenesis,* the growth and development of your brain. When your dentate gyrus is not stimulated, you run a far greater risk of cognitive decline. Remember, you can do this in one stint of 44 minutes or two shorter 22-minute workouts.

## WAKE UP YOUR BRAIN!

### The N-Back

Practice the n-back for 12 minutes a day, going through each level listed below. While a minimum of 12 minutes of the n-back each day is part of the 7-Day Energy Revolution, you will get the best results if you practice the n-back on a regular basis. When it comes to your memory, it's use it or lose it!

*Instructions for Level 1:* Begin with level 1, which starts with the grid on page 237. Notice that one of the nine boxes in the grid contains a shape. Look at the grid for about two seconds and memorize which box contains a shape. (You don't need to memorize the shape itself for now; you'll do that when you move on to level 2.) Next, look at the second grid while covering the first grid with your fingers, an index card, or a piece of paper. Look at this grid for two seconds and memorize which box contains a shape. Then look away.

Now see if you can remember both boxes by reciting your answers, to yourself or out loud, in reverse order. Check to see if you are correct by looking back at the grids. The top right box contains a shape in the first grid and the bottom right box contains a shape in the second grid on page 237, so you would say to yourself, *bottom right,* and then, *top right,* and then check to see if your answers are correct. Eventually, you will notice multiple shapes in the same grid, which will make it even more challenging. Again, just memorize the boxes that contain shapes, not the shapes themselves.

Once you have mastered two grids at a time with mostly correct answers, increase the number of grids you will memorize to three, four, and so on. There is no specific number you need to reach. The goal is to sharpen your brain and increase the number of grids you can memorize correctly.

*Instructions for Level 2:* Once you feel sufficiently challenged, move on to level 2. Follow the same instructions as you did in level 1 with the same grids, but memorize both the box *and* the shape. There is a triangle in the top right box in the first grid and a circle in the bottom right box in the second grid on page 237, so you would say to yourself, *bottom right circle,* and then, *top right triangle,* as you look back to see if you have memorized these correctly. Eventually, there will be more than one shape, which will make it even more challenging.

Once you have mastered two grids at a time with mostly correct answers, increase the number of grids you will memorize to three, four, and so on.

Here is an example of what the grids look like:

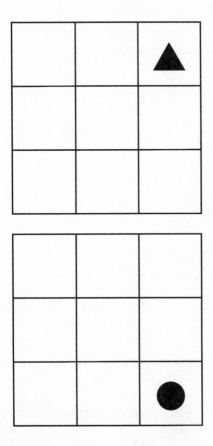

## BRING SOME NOVELTY INTO YOUR LIFE

Every day for the next week, you will try a new activity that stimulates and helps grow your brain. You can come up with your own activities in addition to the ones I suggest on pages 212 through 218, using these guidelines:

- Do something new today that gives you a sense of PLEASURE.

- Do something new today that gives you a sense of PRODUCTIVITY.

- Do something new today that gives you a sense of POWER.

- Do something new today that gives you a sense of PRIDE.

- Do something new today that gives you a sense of PASSION.

- Do something new today that gives you a sense of PEACE.

- Do something new today that gives you a sense of PURPOSE.

## EAT ONE FOOD CONTAINING TURMERIC AND BLACK PEPPER

This includes most curries, or get in the habit of downing my daily wellness shot: Stir a half teaspoon of turmeric and black pepper into an ounce of cold water. If you're feeling particularly brave, add a squeeze of fresh lemon juice and cayenne pepper.

## EXTEND YOUR ATTENTION SPAN

Remember: you can return to all your favorite vices 20 percent of the time once you have completed this week of the program. But for now, I am asking you to cut back on your media use so you can experience the changes in your brain, mood, energy levels, and quality of sleep.

- No TV or watching any sort of entertainment online
- No video games

- No movies except those in a movie theater
- No social media
- Three hours of phone, tablet, and computer-free time during your waking hours, which can be three consecutive hours or three one-hour breaks

Again, after this week, you will be able to reintroduce *moderate* amounts (no more than one hour a day) of television and social media. The key is to recognize how much more clear headed you feel when you have removed or reduced the 24-hour distractions in your life.

## WEEK 3: THE 7-DAY SPIRIT REVOLUTION

In this third and final week of the program, the time has come to move you from aimless and "blah" to inspired, connected, and purposeful.

The focus of this week is on your connections to yourself, your loved ones, and the larger rhythms of the universe. Believe it or not, these are just as important to brain's health as what you eat and how often you exercise! Animals don't need to meditate or pray because they don't have the highly developed part of the brain that makes us uniquely human: the prefrontal cortex. The prefrontal cortex and the hippocampus are where physical changes and neurogenesis can occur. Thus, some form of meditation or prayer that promotes connection and purpose is essential to the human experience. So this week, we'll address two crucial components of brain health that are often overlooked:

1. **Meaning and purpose:** Being in touch with your own unique life's purpose is terrific for your brain.

2. **Feeling connected to something larger than yourself:** This larger connection might be a religious or spiritual practice; an attachment to nature and animals; or a philosophical, political, or scientific awareness of a larger world. However you experience this connection

to something larger, science shows that it is hugely important for brain health. For example, studies of monks who meditate daily reveal distinct improvements in their prefrontal cortex, the part of the brain that makes decisions and controls emotional responses. That's what we're going to start doing for you!

Turn to pages 195 to 233 in the appendix for a day-by-day breakdown of the meditation practices you'll be trying. You will find that just a few minutes a day can transform the way you experience your daily life.

## THE REST OF YOUR LIFE

As I mentioned at the beginning of this chapter, you will want to be really strict, following the guidelines I lay out to the letter, during each week. However, living like this for the rest of your life is pretty much impossible. So just try to do it 80 percent of the time. This flexibility will allow you to maintain the changes you've made for the rest of your life. And whenever you're feeling blah in your mood, energy, or spirit, feel free to come back and repeat one or more of the revolutions.

Repeat the 7-Day Mood Revolution whenever you:

- Feel your mood could use some boosting

- Feel a little too "up and down" and notice the "little things" are getting to you

- Have fallen "off the wagon" in terms of what you're eating and have overindulged in what you eat or drink (e.g., coming back from a vacation or a bachelor party in Vegas)

- Notice you're falling back into old patterns of thinking that prevent you from reaching your potential

- Are going through a difficult time like a breakup or job transition

Repeat the 7-Day Energy Revolution whenever you:

- Notice your energy is off
- Haven't exercised in days
- Feel lazy
- Feel like you're in a rut with more of the "same old"
- Feel like you're not functioning at your full potential
- Are watching too much TV or overindulging in social media
- Aren't sleeping well, at regular times
- Are jet-lagged
- Are having trouble concentrating
- Are in need of some "sharpening"

Repeat the 7-Day Spirit Revolution whenever you:

- Feel disconnected or detached
- Feel frazzled
- Haven't meditated or prayed for days
- Are feeling spiritually thirsty
- Feel the need for more peace
- Feel like you're in a spiritual crisis

And remember, these strategies are not designed to treat diseases or more serious mental illnesses that should be treated by your primary care physician or other health-care professionals. Those with special conditions should consult their doctor before starting this program and modify if needed.

# CHAPTER 17

# Day by Day

In the previous chapter, I laid out the details of what work you'll be doing during each week of the program. In this chapter, I'll go through a quick reminder of the basics and then provide some deeper explanation of the exercises you will do each day. At the beginning of each daily section in the first two weeks, there's an area where you can track the dietary, exercise, sleep, and technology adjustments you're making. Then in the middle you'll find an exercise to do. And finally at the end of each day there's a section to evaluate how you're feeling. In the final week, there are exercises and evaluation sections.

## WORKBOOK FOR WEEK 1:
## THE 7-DAY MOOD REVOLUTION

Remember: No sugar or artificial sweeteners (page 174). No flour or processed snacks (page 176). No foods that are high in pro-inflammatory omega-6s (page 179). No recreational drugs or smoking (page 180). And reduced caffeine and alcohol (page 180). But you will add at least one omega-3 superfood each day (page 181) and seven servings of fruits and vegetables (page 183).

**DAY 1**

## Lifestyle Tracking

Omega-3 superfood (min): __

Seven vegetable and fruit servings (min):
1__ 2__ 3__ 4__ 5__ 6__ 7__

Caffeine (200 mg max): _____

Alcohol (max): 1__

**Exercise: Make a conscious note every time you engage in today's pitfall thought pattern of the day: *Personalization*.** Remember that by paying attention you'll start to notice how often this thought pattern shows up in your life. Try to remember specific instances of experiencing this thought pattern because, at the end of the day, I'll ask you to evaluate how personalization affects your life.

Personalization is taking something negative that is happening in your life and pinning all the blame on yourself. You go to a job interview and don't get the job; you tell yourself you're not smart enough. The person you went on a date with doesn't call you back; you tell yourself you're not attractive enough.

The opposite of personalization is to place more blame for negative events on causes outside of yourself. This latter way of looking at things has been linked to confidence and optimism.

While there are times in life when it's necessary to address deficits and strive for self-improvement, most of the time there are countless alternative explanations that help explain why something didn't go your way. And most people err on the side of blaming themselves *too* much when the alternative explanation is actually the objective reality of what happened.

By choosing to blame yourself, you create a self-fulfilling prophecy. Personalization robs you of self-worth and confidence, and this affects future choices in a negative way, leading to more negative outcomes. The fact is, you probably didn't get the job because the boss's son-in-law got hired. She didn't call you back because she's still in love with her ex.

The one time you should internalize and take the credit? When something *does* go your way. I got the second interview because I'm personable and intelligent. My spouse is married to me because I'm kind and beautiful.

Notice each time you catch yourself using this pitfall thought pattern today.

## End-of-Day Evaluation

How am I feeling today (mood), with 10 being the best?
1 2 3 4 5 6 7 8 9 10

How am I thinking today (focus and attention), with 10 being the best?
1 2 3 4 5 6 7 8 9 10

How is my energy level today, with 10 being the best?
1 2 3 4 5 6 7 8 9 10

Recall all the times you noticed yourself engaging in personalization today. Now take a moment to reflect on how you would think and feel if you didn't engage in this pitfall thought pattern. Ask yourself the following questions:

- How differently would I feel if I considered alternative explanations in which I don't blame myself for things not going my way?

- How differently would I feel if I took the credit for the things that do go my way?

- If I changed this pitfall thought pattern, how would it change the way I feel?

- If I changed this pitfall thought pattern, how would this change my life?

## Lifestyle Tracking

Omega-3 superfood (min): __

Seven vegetable and fruit servings (min):
1__ 2__ 3__ 4__ 5__ 6__ 7__

Caffeine (200 mg max): _____

Alcohol (max): 1__

**Exercise: Make a conscious note every time you engage in today's pitfall thought pattern of the day: *Pervasiveness*.** Remember that by paying attention you'll start to notice how often this thought pattern shows up in your life. Try to remember specific instances of experiencing this thought pattern because, at the end of the day, I'll ask you to evaluate how pervasiveness affects your life.

Pervasiveness means allowing problems in one area of your life to bleed into other areas of your life. You are having problems at work, so you take your stress out on your significant other. Or your love life is a mess and you haven't yet fully recovered from your divorce, so you perceive your whole life as one big failure. When you allow failure in one area of your life to mean your whole life is a failure, it affects not only your well-being but also your self-worth.

It's easy to let pervasiveness in, but the problem with this is that you should rely on your strengths to buoy you up instead of letting an isolated problem drag your entire life down. Consider the opposite: you allow strengths and successes in one area of your life to brighten every area of your life.

Imagine you're a ship sailing across the Atlantic Ocean. If there's a leak in one part of the ship, seal that part off. By doing so, you'll still float and will effortlessly make the journey. That leak will get fixed this week or next month, but in the meantime you'll still be floating. Rely on the other parts (e.g., the strengths in your life) to keep you floating. What you *don't* want to do is to allow that leak to spread through the entire ship, because then the ship goes down.

## End-of-Day Evaluation

How am I feeling today (mood), with 10 being the best?
1  2  3  4  5  6  7  8  9  10

How am I thinking today (focus and attention), with 10 being the best?
1  2  3  4  5  6  7  8  9  10

How is my energy level today, with 10 being the best?
1  2  3  4  5  6  7  8  9  10

Recall all the times you noticed yourself engaging in pervasiveness today. Now take a moment to reflect on how you would think and feel if you didn't engage in this pitfall thought pattern. Ask yourself the following questions:

- How differently would I feel if I allowed everything going right in my life to lift me up?

- What would change if I didn't get bogged down by the things in my life that I'm struggling with for right now?

- If I changed this pitfall thought pattern, how would it change the way I feel?

- If I changed this pitfall thought pattern, how would this change my life?

## Lifestyle Tracking

Omega-3 superfood (min): __

Seven vegetable and fruit servings (min):
1__ 2__ 3__ 4__ 5__ 6__ 7__

Caffeine (200 mg max): _____

Alcohol (max): 1__

**Exercise: Make a conscious note every time you engage in today's pitfall thought pattern of the day: *Paralysis-analysis*.** Remember that by paying attention you'll start to notice how often this thought pattern shows up in your life. Try to remember specific instances of experiencing this thought pattern because, at the end of the day, I'll ask you to evaluate how paralysis-analysis affects your life.

Paralysis-analysis is a thought pattern marked by excess worry and rumination, which make it difficult or impossible to move forward in your life. When a fearful thought or feeling enters your awareness, you ruminate, stew, and overanalyze the situation. By turning the negative thought over in your mind again and again, you become fearful and this can create a state of paralysis.

Notice how worry does nothing to change a situation. While it's necessary to give problems some amount of thought, you can't think yourself out of most negative situations. In weeks 2 and 3 of the program, you'll learn powerful antidotes to paralysis-analysis: filling your life with purposeful action and mindfulness of thoughts, respectively. But the first step is what you will do today as you become aware of this pitfall thought pattern and the way it holds you back. By doing so, you are beginning to take its power away.

## End-of-Day Evaluation

How am I feeling today (mood), with 10 being the best?
1 2 3 4 5 6 7 8 9 10

How am I thinking today (focus and attention), with 10 being the best?
1 2 3 4 5 6 7 8 9 10

How is my energy level today, with 10 being the best?
1 2 3 4 5 6 7 8 9 10

Recall all the times you noticed yourself engaging in paralysis-analysis today. Now take a moment to reflect on how you would think and feel if you didn't engage in this pitfall thought pattern. Ask yourself the following questions:

- How differently would I feel if I didn't engage in the overanalysis of worries that has paralyzed me with fear?

- What could I be doing right now if I wasn't ruminating and took action instead?

- If I changed this pitfall thought pattern, how would it change the way I feel?

- If I changed this pitfall thought pattern, how would this change my life?

## Lifestyle Tracking

Omega-3 superfood (min): __

Seven vegetable and fruit servings (min):
1__ 2__ 3__ 4__ 5__ 6__ 7__

Caffeine (200 mg max): _____

Alcohol (max): 1__

**Exercise: Make a conscious note every time you engage in today's pitfall thought pattern of the day:** *Pessimism.* Remember that by paying attention you'll start to notice how often this thought pattern shows up in your life. Try to remember specific instances of experiencing this thought pattern because, at the end of the day, I'll ask you to evaluate how pessimism affects your life.

Pessimism means you look for what's wrong in your life instead of focusing on what's right. You're always worrying about the possible worst-case-scenario outcome instead of the more probable, favorable one. Or you're focusing on the catastrophic scenario instead of seeing positive, optimistic outcomes.

This pitfall thought pattern actually creates self-fulfilling prophecies where your energy makes negative outcomes more probable. To some degree, looking on the bright side is a choice. Everyone has both blessings and burdens in their lives. Today, choose to focus on the blessings. Remember the mantra "There is no way to happiness; happiness is the way."

You may not be exactly where you thought you'd be in your life, but there are probably some accomplishments that you're really proud of. Remember the compliments. Meditate on the phrase "Today, I'm exactly where I should be, because that's exactly where I am."

Pessimism prevents you from seeing the blessings you already have in your life; optimism makes every day a little sunnier and attracts an abundance of even more blessings.

## End-of-Day Evaluation

How am I feeling today (mood), with 10 being the best?
1 2 3 4 5 6 7 8 9 10

How am I thinking today (focus and attention), with 10 being the best?
1 2 3 4 5 6 7 8 9 10

How is my energy level today, with 10 being the best?
1 2 3 4 5 6 7 8 9 10

Recall all the times you noticed yourself engaging in pessimistic thinking today. Now take a moment to reflect on how you would think and feel if you didn't engage in this pitfall thought pattern. Ask yourself the following questions:

- How differently would I feel if I started to look for what's right in my life instead of what's wrong?

- How would optimism invite gratitude into my life and create even more abundance?

- If I changed this pitfall thought pattern, how would it change the way I feel?

- If I changed this pitfall thought pattern, how would this change my life?

## Lifestyle Tracking

Omega-3 superfood (min): __

Seven vegetable and fruit servings (min):
1__ 2__ 3__ 4__ 5__ 6__ 7__

Caffeine (200 mg max): _____

Alcohol (max): 1__

**Exercise: Make a conscious note every time you engage in today's pitfall thought pattern of the day:** *Polarization.* Remember that by paying attention you'll start to notice how often this thought pattern shows up in your life. Try to remember specific instances of experiencing this thought pattern because, at the end of the day, I'll ask you to evaluate how polarization affects your life.

Polarization means that you are seeing the world through a black-or-white, on-or-off lens without considering solutions that reside in the shades of gray that lie between black and white. You consider one option "right" and the other "wrong." This also means that if something isn't working perfectly, you perceive it as not working at all. An A- becomes an F. This pitfall thought pattern often leads to perfectionism and trying to control everything in your life . . . or needing to control one thing when so many other things feel out of control.

By engaging in this pitfall thought pattern, you limit the possibilities in your life. You also may be missing out on seeing the world through someone else's lens and in doing so, helping them feel seen and heard, which creates intimacy and connection.

Being laid off or coming to the end of a relationship isn't a failure; it's an opportunity to ask, "What did I learn from this experience?" Having a fight with your significant other isn't about figuring out who's right and who's wrong; it's about understanding what part *does* make sense about his or her point of view and what it says about what he or she needs. Polarization makes it difficult to perceive blessings since you ignore the 99 other possible answers while being obsessed with just one.

## End-of-Day Evaluation

How am I feeling today (mood), with 10 being the best?
1 2 3 4 5 6 7 8 9 10

How am I thinking today (focus and attention), with 10 being the best?
1 2 3 4 5 6 7 8 9 10

How is my energy level today, with 10 being the best?
1 2 3 4 5 6 7 8 9 10

Recall all the times you noticed yourself engaging in polarized thinking today. Now take a moment to reflect on how you would think and feel if you didn't engage in this pitfall thought pattern. Ask yourself the following questions:

- How would looking for more "gray area" and less "black or white" in thinking and action help me move through the world with more grace?

- How would this help me invite equanimity into my life?

- If I changed this pitfall thought pattern, how would it change the way I feel?

- If I changed this pitfall thought pattern, how would this change my life?

DAY 6

## Lifestyle Tracking

Omega-3 superfood (min): __

Seven vegetable and fruit servings (min):
1__ 2__ 3__ 4__ 5__ 6__ 7__

Caffeine (200 mg max): _____

Alcohol (max): 1__

**Exercise: Make a conscious note every time you engage in today's pitfall thought pattern of the day:** *Psychic.* Remember that by paying attention you'll start to notice how often this thought pattern shows up in your life. Try to remember specific instances of experiencing this thought pattern because, at the end of the day, I'll ask you to evaluate how psychic thinking affects your life.

Psychic is a thought pattern in which you expect others to read your mind without verbalizing exactly what you're feeling, thinking, or needing. You expect others to interpret your behavior or facial expressions, and when they don't do so, you become hurt or angry. In addition to expecting others to be psychic, you also believe *you* are psychic; when you make negative assumptions about the future without ever having the experience, you are predicting the future.

When you're upset about something your significant other did, stomping around the house and taking on a curt tone of voice only makes things worse. Most of the time, this person needs you to explain what exactly hurt you *and* to ask for what you do need, in positive and specific language.

Or perhaps you're single. If you've made psychic predictions that the person you like will decline your dinner invitation if you ask him or her out—and then don't actually extend the invitation—your psychic thinking has blocked any possibility for the event to occur. Yes, you *may* have been hurt. But you may have been pleasantly surprised. It's up to you to take risks if you are seeking great rewards.

By engaging in this pitfall thought pattern, you block miracles from occurring. By not letting it go, you prevent intimacy and growth in relationships and within yourself.

## End-of-Day Evaluation

How am I feeling today (mood), with 10 being the best?
1 2 3 4 5 6 7 8 9 10

How am I thinking today (focus and attention), with 10 being the best?
1 2 3 4 5 6 7 8 9 10

How is my energy level today, with 10 being the best?
1 2 3 4 5 6 7 8 9 10

Recall all the times you noticed yourself engaging in psychic thinking today. Now take a moment to reflect on how you would think and feel if you didn't engage in this pitfall thought pattern. Ask yourself the following questions:

- If I ask for exactly what I need from others, how will this change my relationships?

- If I take a risk by sharing my own feelings while asking the same of others, how will this help me see what life could have in store for me?

- If I changed this pitfall thought pattern, how would it change the way I feel?

- If I changed this pitfall thought pattern, how would this change my life?

## Lifestyle Tracking

Omega-3 superfood (min): __

Seven vegetable and fruit servings (min):
1__ 2__ 3__ 4__ 5__ 6__ 7__

Caffeine (200 mg max): _____

Alcohol (max): 1__

**Exercise: Make a conscious note every time you engage in today's pitfall thought pattern of the day:** *Permanence.* Remember that by paying attention you'll start to notice how often this thought pattern shows up in your life. Try to remember specific instances of experiencing this thought pattern because, at the end of the day, I'll ask you to evaluate how permanence affects your life.

Permanence means that you feel like a current negative situation will never change. When you're in a bad mood or stressed out, it *feels* like it's always been this way and always *will be* this way. Even in times when you *logically* know "this too shall pass," *emotionally* it feels like the sadness, anxiety, or situation will never end.

This phenomenon has to do with mood-congruent recall in the brain. This means that when you're sad, all the sad memories "light up" in the brain while happy memories fade. Of course, this contributes to that feeling that your life has always been, is now, and always will be sad. Remember, however, that this is only a temporary illusion and not objective reality.

Consider the opposite of this point of view: negative events and feeling states are temporary. Do you have evidence of this? Can you remember a situation many years ago—a relationship ending or facing a disappointment in your career—where it felt like the black cloud would never clear . . . but then it did? And if you remembered that negative feeling states are temporary, would this help you to bounce back faster?

Imagine how this would transform your energy and mood. And underneath this way of thinking is a core belief that the universe, human beings, and life itself are inherently good. Because if this is true, then "bad" will eventually always give way to "good." By thinking in this alternate way, you invite more faith into your life.

## End-of-Day Evaluation

How am I feeling today (mood), with 10 being the best?
1 2 3 4 5 6 7 8 9 10

How am I thinking today (focus and attention), with 10 being the best?
1 2 3 4 5 6 7 8 9 10

How is my energy level today, with 10 being the best?
1 2 3 4 5 6 7 8 9 10

Recall all the times you noticed yourself engaging in permanence today. Now take a moment to reflect on how you would think and feel if you didn't engage in this pitfall thought pattern. Ask yourself the following questions:

- How would I feel if I remembered the adage "This, too, shall pass"?

- If I allow the logical part of me that knows that storm clouds pass to overrule the emotional part of me that is stuck in negative emotion, how would I invite more joy, faith, and peace into my life?

- If I changed this pitfall thought pattern, how would it change the way I feel?

- If I changed this pitfall thought pattern, how would this change my life?

## WORKBOOK FOR WEEK 2:
## THE 7-DAY ENERGY REVOLUTION

Remember: Get 7.5 to 8.5 hours of sleep each night (page 186). Get moving with 44 minutes of exercise a day (page 187). Wake up your brain with 12 minutes of the n-back tests (page 187). Eat one food containing turmeric and black pepper each day (page 190). Extend your attention span with some technology-use changes (page 190). Bring some novelty into your life with some sense-focused exercises (page 189). After you do these exercises, take a moment to concentrate on how you feel because of what you just did. At the end of each day, I'll walk you through some questions that will help you get even more out of the experience.

**DAY 8**

## Lifestyle Tracking

Turmeric superfood: ___

N-back (min 12 minutes): _____

Exercise (min 44 minutes in one or two sessions): 22_____ 44_____

Three waking hours with no TV, computer, phone, or tablet: 1__ 2__ 3__

Bedtime: _____

Wake up: _____

## Exercise: Novelty of the day: *PLEASURE*

Do something new or novel today that you find pleasurable. It can be something small like lighting a candle with a new aroma. Go to a restaurant you've been wanting to try. Taste a new gelato flavor. Visit a beach or lake you've never been to before.

## End-of-Day Evaluation

How am I feeling today (mood), with 10 being the best?
1 2 3 4 5 6 7 8 9 10

How am I thinking today (focus and attention), with 10 being the best?
1 2 3 4 5 6 7 8 9 10

How is my energy level today, with 10 being the best?
1 2 3 4 5 6 7 8 9 10

How did engaging in an activity that brought me pleasure change my mood today? If I continued to make a conscious effort to engage in more activities like this, how would it change my life?

## Lifestyle Tracking

Turmeric superfood: __

N-back (min 12 minutes): ____

Exercise (min 44 minutes in one or two sessions): 22____ 44____

Three waking hours with no TV, computer, phone, or tablet: 1__ 2__ 3__

Bedtime: ____

Wake up: ____

## Exercise: Novelty of the day: *PRODUCTIVITY*

Do something new or novel today that is productive. Clean out that garage for the first time. Rearrange the furniture in your living room. Drop off your dry cleaning at an environmentally friendly dry cleaner. Buy an air-cleaning plant for your home. Go to a class at the gym you've never been to before. Clean out your closet and drop the clothes off at a charity.

## End-of-Day Evaluation

How am I feeling today (mood), with 10 being the best?
1 2 3 4 5 6 7 8 9 10

How am I thinking today (focus and attention), with 10 being the best?
1 2 3 4 5 6 7 8 9 10

How is my energy level today, with 10 being the best?
1 2 3 4 5 6 7 8 9 10

How did engaging in a productive activity change my mood today? If I continued to make a conscious effort to engage in more activities like this, how would it change my life?

**DAY 10**

## Lifestyle Tracking

Turmeric superfood: __

N-back (min 12 minutes): ____

Exercise (min 44 minutes in one or two sessions): 22____ 44____

Three waking hours with no TV, computer, phone, or tablet: 1__ 2__ 3__

Bedtime: ____

Wake up: ____

## Exercise: Novelty of the day: *POWER*

Do something new or novel today that makes you feel powerful. Lift weights for the first time. If you're a good writer, start writing that blog or script you've been meaning to start. If you're looking for a new job, redo your résumé and send it to places you hadn't previously considered. If you're shy, take a class and sit at the front. See how it feels to try on this new sense of power in your life and how it can create abundance.

## End-of-Day Evaluation

How am I feeling today (mood), with 10 being the best?
1 2 3 4 5 6 7 8 9 10

How am I thinking today (focus and attention), with 10 being the best?
1 2 3 4 5 6 7 8 9 10

How is my energy level today, with 10 being the best?
1 2 3 4 5 6 7 8 9 10

How did engaging in an activity that made me feel powerful change my mood today? If I continued to make a conscious effort to engage in more activities like this, how would it change my life?

## Lifestyle Tracking

Turmeric superfood: __

N-back (min 12 minutes): ____

Exercise (min 44 minutes in one or two sessions): 22____ 44____

Three waking hours with no TV, computer, phone, or tablet: 1__ 2__ 3__

Bedtime: ____

Wake up: ____

## Exercise: Novelty of the day: *PRIDE*

Do something new or novel today that makes you feel proud. If you're a great cook, invite some friends over to sample your latest culinary creation. If you're proud of your way with dogs, volunteer with a rescue group to walk them. Focus on your strengths and remember how great it is to be proud of what you do and who you are.

## End-of-Day Evaluation

How am I feeling today (mood), with 10 being the best?
1 2 3 4 5 6 7 8 9 10

How am I thinking today (focus and attention), with 10 being the best?
1 2 3 4 5 6 7 8 9 10

How is my energy level today, with 10 being the best?
1 2 3 4 5 6 7 8 9 10

How did engaging in an activity that makes me feel proud change my mood today? If I continued to make a conscious effort to engage in more activities like this, how would it change my life?

## Lifestyle Tracking

Turmeric superfood: __

N-back (min 12 minutes): ____

Exercise (min 44 minutes in one or two sessions): 22____ 44____

Three waking hours with no TV, computer, phone, or tablet: 1__ 2__ 3__

Bedtime: ____

Wake up: ____

## Exercise: Novelty of the day: *PASSION*

Do something new or novel today that reminds you of what you're truly passionate about. If you used to love dancing, go to a dance class. If you're passionate about art, go to a museum or exhibit you haven't been to. Infuse your life with activities that help you remind you of your passions, and you'll change your attention and remember who you are.

## End-of-Day Evaluation

How am I feeling today (mood), with 10 being the best?
1 2 3 4 5 6 7 8 9 10

How am I thinking today (focus and attention), with 10 being the best?
1 2 3 4 5 6 7 8 9 10

How is my energy level today, with 10 being the best?
1 2 3 4 5 6 7 8 9 10

How did engaging in an activity that I'm passionate about change my mood today? If I continued to make a conscious effort to engage in more activities like this, how would it change my life?

## Lifestyle Tracking

Turmeric superfood: __

N-back (min 12 minutes): ____

Exercise (min 44 minutes in one or two sessions): 22____ 44____

Three waking hours with no TV, computer, phone, or tablet: 1__ 2__ 3__

Bedtime: ____

Wake up: ____

## Exercise: Novelty of the day: *PEACE*

Do something new or novel today that gives you a sense of peace. Go to a park or on a hike you've never been to before, and marvel at the beauty of nature. Try a yoga class you've never been to before. Play a new song, and hear it with every bone in your body. Remember that you always have the opportunity to cultivate a sense of peace by choosing what to do with your mind and body.

## Evaluation

How am I feeling today (mood), with 10 being the best?
1 2 3 4 5 6 7 8 9 10

How am I thinking today (focus and attention), with 10 being the best?
1 2 3 4 5 6 7 8 9 10

How is my energy level today, with 10 being the best?
1 2 3 4 5 6 7 8 9 10

How did engaging in an activity that brought me peace change my mood today? If I continued to make a conscious effort to engage in more activities like this, how would it change my life?

## Lifestyle Tracking

Turmeric superfood: __

N-back (min 12 minutes): ____

Exercise (min 44 minutes in one or two sessions): 22____ 44____

Three waking hours with no TV, computer, phone, or tablet: 1__ 2__ 3__

Bedtime: ____

Wake up: ____

## Exercise: Novelty of the day: *PURPOSE*

Do something new or novel today that gives you a sense of purpose. If you've been considering adoption, go to the library and read a book on it. If your kids mean everything to you, buy them a thoughtful gift or write them a heartfelt note. If faith has been absent in your life for a while, find a place to meditate or pray. If you'd like to volunteer more, take a concrete step today in making that a reality. Remember that filling your days with a sense of purpose is paramount to leading a happy, meaningful life.

## Evaluation

How am I feeling today (mood), with 10 being the best?
1 2 3 4 5 6 7 8 9 10

How am I thinking today (focus and attention), with 10 being the best?
1 2 3 4 5 6 7 8 9 10

How is my energy level today, with 10 being the best?
1 2 3 4 5 6 7 8 9 10

How did engaging in an activity that brought me a sense of purpose change my mood today? If I continued to make a conscious effort to engage in more activities like this, how would it change my life?

## WORKBOOK FOR WEEK 3:
## THE 7-DAY SPIRIT REVOLUTION

Remember: this week is all about your spirit, so we'll enrich this part of who you are by starting each day with a spiritual exercise that you can take with you as you go about your day. This spiritual exercise may include a few tasks or it may simply involve you setting an intention.

You will also find a 12-minute meditation to do each day. Complete this meditation practice at any point during your day. Find a quiet and comfortable place where you won't be disturbed. First, read the meditation a few times so you know exactly what is expected of you. Then, set a timer for 12 minutes. Begin by closing your eyes. Then walk yourself through the meditation in your mind. If you finish the instructions before the timer goes off, rest in the mindful silence you have cultivated and relish the beauty of the moment. If the timer goes off and you haven't completed the practice yet—or if you find yourself wanting to meditate for more than 12 minutes—take all the time you need or want.

After you finish each spiritual exercise and meditation during this week, take a moment to think about what you learned, how you felt, or what you observed during the practice. At the end of each day, I'll lead you through some specific questions to ask yourself about your experience with these exercises.

## Spiritual Exercise: *The Half Smile*

Putting a half smile on your face causes a neurochemical response that helps you link into the feedback loop of happiness. When you are happy, you tend to smile. But it also works in reverse: if you smile, you tend to feel happier.

So for today, try to put a half smile in everything you do. Half smile when you wake up groggy. Half smile when you're stuck in traffic. Half smile when you're on the treadmill. Half smile when you're in a stressful meeting. Half smile when you're tired. See how this simple act can have a profound effect on the way you feel. See how this outside-in approach elicits feelings of gratitude, happiness, and peace.

## 12-Minute Meditation: *The Flashlight*

Set your timer for 12 minutes. Lie down on the floor or your bed. Close your eyes. For 12 minutes, you're going to put your attention on the smallest sensation you're experiencing in your body. Imagine you're holding a flashlight and are going to take 12 minutes to shine the light from your head to your toes, and this "flashlight" represents your awareness.

Start with your scalp, and see if you can actually feel the weight of your hair. Sense every follicle as you move down and feel the place where your forehead meets your hairline or scalp. Keep scanning down your nose, eyelashes, and eyebrows, and move slowly throughout your entire body. As the light scans different parts of your body, allow it to relax that part as well. But remember: this practice is not about falling asleep. It's about falling "awake."

Whenever a thought comes into your consciousness and is trying to take some of the light away from your body, just notice it gently. It's probably going to happen tens or hundreds of times throughout these 12 minutes, and that's okay. Whenever it happens, just bring the light of your awareness back to wherever you left off without any sort of judgment. Notice what it's like to actually *feel* your body. Notice that you have millions of sensations to pay attention to just from your skin cells or the place where your back makes contact with your bed.

In the last moments of this meditation, see if you have that sensation of actually *being in your body*. Quietly say to yourself, *Ahhhh . . . Here I am. The part of me that's separate from what I do or what I think. Here I am in the present moment. Here I am in my body.*

## End-of-Day Evaluation

How am I feeling today (mood), with 10 being the best?
1 2 3 4 5 6 7 8 9 10

How am I thinking today (focus and attention), with 10 being the best?
1 2 3 4 5 6 7 8 9 10

How is my energy level today, with 10 being the best?
1 2 3 4 5 6 7 8 9 10

How did the half smile transform my day today? If I began to live my life with a half smile, what would change? How did the flashlight meditation help me feel more mindful of the present moment? How did it help me to feel like I'm "in" my body? What was one spiritual lesson I learned through these practices today?

## Spiritual Exercise: *"What's Right?"*

At least once an hour, take note of something pleasant. It could be a thought, a sensation, or a feeling. Maybe you notice a bird chirping, and you take a moment to stop and sense that pleasant sound. You finish a task at work, and you consciously recognize that feeling of accomplishment. And with it, you notice the self-worth and happiness that's attached to it. You take note that you're feeling pretty peaceful right now. Just soak that in and let it land on you.

This exercise helps change your selective attention. Look around the room right now and say to yourself, *Green. Green. Green.* Your eye will go to all of the green things in the room, even though nothing in the room actually changed color; there's the same amount of green there was just a moment ago.

And so it goes with what you choose to pay attention to. Just as you can look around the room and say *green,* you can look around your life and say to yourself, *What's right, what's right, what's right?* You have the power to change your subjective experience of the present moment by choosing to pay attention to the pleasant or positive attributes instead of the negative or unpleasant ones. And the more you learn to notice and appreciate the most subtle of pleasant experiences in your life, the more you'll find them . . . and the less miserable you will be as you stop telling yourself, *I'll be happy when* _____ .

There is no way to happiness. Happiness is the way.

## 12-Minute Meditation: *Sound Meditation*

Put on a piece of uplifting or soothing music that you'll listen to for the next 12 minutes. Lie down on your bed or the floor. Close your eyes.

Hear the music in an entirely different way than you've ever heard music before. Instead of just hearing it with your ears while concurrently daydreaming or half hearing, hear this piece of music with your entire body.

Hear the music with your skin. Hear it with your bones. Hear it with your fingers. Hear it with your toes.

See if you can perceive the spaces between the bass notes or lyrics. See if you can feel the actual moment when the note lands on your skin.

## End-of-Day Evaluation

How am I feeling today (mood), with 10 being the best?
1 2 3 4 5 6 7 8 9 10

How am I thinking today (focus and attention), with 10 being the best?
1 2 3 4 5 6 7 8 9 10

How is my energy level today, with 10 being the best?
1 2 3 4 5 6 7 8 9 10

How did looking for the "what's right" transform my day today? How does this help me invite more gratitude into my daily life? How did the sound meditation help invite more present-mindedness to all things I do? If I did this on a regular basis, how would it change my life? What was one spiritual lesson I learned through these practices today?

## Spiritual Exercise: *One Thing at a Time*

Today, set an intention to do one thing *and only one thing* at a time. When you're washing the dishes, give the action your full attention and really wash the dishes. When you're taking a shower, feel every drop of water. Notice sensations you've been taking for granted that happen each and every day.

When you're walking from your car to your office, just walk. Give it all your attention, and see things that you've been taking for granted. Feel the air on your cheek and the sunlight on your face. When you're driving, drive. Notice trees or shops you've never noticed. When you're working, work. If something comes up that tries to take you away from what you're doing—like daydreaming or worrying—then give *that* your full attention for a moment or two until it runs its course. But do it mindfully, which means be cognizant of the fact that you're doing it. Oftentimes, we're daydreaming without even *realizing* we're doing it! Then come back to whatever you were doing, and do that.

See what it's like to do just one thing at a time.

## 12-Minute Meditation: *Kirtan Kriya*

This meditation is particularly effective for preserving memory and can even reverse memory loss. It's an active meditation that requires you to use your fingers and, yes, your singing voice while you meditate.

You will sing the four sounds *Sa, Ta, Na, Ma* over and over again to the first four notes of "Mary Had a Little Lamb." Replace "Mar-y had a . . ." with "Sa, Ta, Na, Ma . . ."

When you sing *Sa,* touch your thumbs to your index fingers.

When you sing *Ta,* touch your thumbs to your middle fingers.

When you sing *Na,* touch your thumbs to your ring fingers.

When you sing *Ma,* touch your thumbs to your pinky fingers.

Repeat. The pace should be about one second per sound. Take a breath after the fourth sound.

For the first two minutes or so, sing in a normal singing voice.

For the next two minutes or so, sing in a whisper.

For the next four minutes or so, sing silently to yourself.

For the next two minutes or so, sing in a whisper again.

For the final two minutes or so, sing in a normal singing voice.

Don't worry about watching the clock to transition exactly to the next stage exactly at the two- or four-minute mark. It's better to keep your eyes closed throughout the meditation practice. If you find the 12-minute timer going off before you have finished the last stage, you can either keep going or stop and adjust your timing the next time you decide to practice this meditation.

You can improve your memory even if you decide to use this meditation in a nonspiritual way. But if you'd like to attach spiritual significance to this practice, you'll reap even more benefits in the form of peace and a feeling of connectivity. This meditation has been used for thousands of years in the kundalini yoga tradition. *Sa* signifies birth and the totality of life. *Ta* is life. *Na* is death and the transformation of consciousness. *Ma* is rebirth and resurrection. Feel connected to the divine and eternal movement of the universe.

## End-of-Day Evaluation

How am I feeling today (mood), with 10 being the best?
1 2 3 4 5 6 7 8 9 10

How am I thinking today (focus and attention), with 10 being the best?
1 2 3 4 5 6 7 8 9 10

How is my energy level today, with 10 being the best?
1 2 3 4 5 6 7 8 9 10

How differently would I feel—how much less frantic and more peaceful—if I invited more doing just "one thing at a time" into my life? Speaking of "only one thing," how would my experience of eating every meal change if I brought a little bit of the mindfulness I cultivated in this meditation into every meal? How can I invite this sense of presence into every act in my life? What was one spiritual lesson I learned through these practices today?

## Spiritual Exercise: *Your Daily Mantra*

Without knowing it, we often go through the world silently repeating a mantra to ourselves and we experience the world through the lens of this mantra. If we have been abused or used, perhaps that mantra is "People hurt me." If we have been abandoned, it can be "People leave." If we are anxious, it's some version of "I'm not okay." If we are depressed or struggle with low self-worth, it's some version of "I'm not good enough," or "There's something wrong with me." The problem is that, through selective attention, we go through our lives looking for evidence of this mantra. And when we look for the evidence to support something, good or bad, we can usually find it.

Today, choose a different mantra. It can be a word or a phrase. Here are some examples:

- "I'm okay."
- "Peace"
- "Equanimity"
- "Patience"
- "I'm good enough."

- "I'm lovable."
- "Loved"
- "People who are right for me *do* stay."
- "One"
- "Love"

Go through your day and see how silently carrying this mantra around affects your experience. See how it can change your interactions with people like co-workers or even strangers. How does it affect your feelings? How does it affect your thoughts?

## 12-Minute Meditation: *The Thought Stream*

Imagine yourself sitting by the side of a peaceful river. The river represents the thoughts and feelings in your mind. For the next 12 minutes, spend some time just watching what's in your river at this moment. Without any judgment . . . without trying to slow the river down or speed it up . . . just watch your river.

And while you're at it, notice the difference between *you* sitting next to the river and the *river* itself. Most of the time, we have a tendency to overidentify with our thoughts and feelings. We believe that we are our thoughts and feelings, and we forget who we are. But we're so much *more* than our thoughts. Feelings come and feelings go. They're useful information to help guide our lives. But we also must remember who we are and not feel imprisoned by them.

This happens when we proverbially *jump into* our river. When you notice you've "jumped in," simply find your way out of the river and feel yourself back on the side of the bank.

You'll be left with the feeling of peace when you sense that part of you that is you. It's the part of you that always has been and always will be. It's the part of you that is connected to all living beings.

## End-of-Day Evaluation

How am I feeling today (mood), with 10 being the best?
1 2 3 4 5 6 7 8 9 10

How am I thinking today (focus and attention), with 10 being the best?
1 2 3 4 5 6 7 8 9 10

How is my energy level today, with 10 being the best?
1 2 3 4 5 6 7 8 9 10

How differently would I feel if I had a more positive daily mantra each and every day? How would this begin to change the way I am in the world? From what I learned during the meditation, how would my life be different if I remembered who I am? How would my relationship to my thoughts and feelings change if I remembered that we are not one and the same? If I started to use them as guides and not as my jailer, how would this change my life? What was one spiritual lesson I learned today through these practices?

## Spiritual Exercise: *Random Acts*

Commit random acts of kindness today. They can be big or they can be small. Start with making eye contact and saying hello to people instead of being glued to your phone, since your presence is one of the greatest gifts you can give to another. It tells them: You matter.

Hold the door for people. Send an e-mail, text, or handwritten note to a friend just telling them what qualities you appreciate about them. Submit an application to volunteer for an organization. Compliment a stranger. Make an online donation to a charity. Buy a meal for a homeless person. Pay for the person behind you at the toll booth. Buy a gift for someone.

## 12-Minute Meditation: *The Loving-Kindness Meditation*

Begin by closing your eyes. Over the next 12 minutes, imagine that the love from your heart actually radiates outward like the circular ripples when a pebble is dropped in a lake.

Start with yourself, and say, *May I be happy and peaceful.* See yourself bathed in your love, which you can visualize as a color, if you'd like.

Then visualize one person who is very close to your heart. Say to yourself, *May this person be happy and peaceful.* See them bathed in your love and compassion.

As the love continues to radiate outward, it includes all your loved ones. Say, *May all my loved ones be happy and peaceful.* The love from your heart grows. Visualize it; see it.

Your loving-kindness is growing so much, it now even includes people you've had disagreements with or who have hurt you. Visualize those people and say, *May they be happy and peaceful.* Notice what it feels like to try on this energy, even if it's just for this moment and this is still something you're working on.

Finally, this loving-kindness grows and includes all beings on the face of the planet. You say, *May all beings be happy and peaceful.*

Sit for a moment and see how the loving-kindness in your heart has the power to reach the entire world. Sit with the feeling that you get from this practice.

## End-of-Day Evaluation

How am I feeling today (mood), with 10 being the best?
1 2 3 4 5 6 7 8 9 10

How am I thinking today (focus and attention), with 10 being the best?
1 2 3 4 5 6 7 8 9 10

How is my energy level today, with 10 being the best?
1 2 3 4 5 6 7 8 9 10

How did committing small acts of kindness today change the way I feel? If I continued to look for opportunities to commit random acts of kindness, how would this change my life? From what I learned during the meditation, how would my life change if I bathed myself and others in an energy of perpetual loving-kindness? What was one spiritual lesson I learned from these practices today?

## Spiritual Exercise: *The Thank-You Note*

Take a moment to write a heartfelt letter to someone who has touched your life in a meaningful way. The person can be in your life now or someone from your past. The person can be living or someone who has passed away.

Write in a positive and specific way about how this person has changed you. How did this experience shape who you are today? Express your heartfelt gratitude to this person.

Send the note if you wish, or keep it as a reminder of this profound gift.

## 12-Minute Meditation:
## *The Examen (Based on St. Ignatius's "Daily Examen")*

This is one of the few meditations that is best to do at the end of your day, so try to schedule 12 free minutes before you get into bed for the night. During those 12 minutes, we will slowly work our way through your connection with the divine and how that expresses itself in your life. Close your eyes as you begin to divert your attention away from the physical and logical parts of who you are. Attune to your spirit and your soul as you walk yourself through this meditation.

First, become aware of the presence of your higher self or God within you. Sit in this profound awareness for a few minutes.

Second, consciously review your day with a sense of gratitude. With a half smile on your face, remember all the joys you have experienced over the course of the day in the presence of your higher self or God. Be thankful for all of the blessings you have received. Quietly sit in this gratitude for a few minutes.

Third, review your emotions. Reflect on the feelings you've experienced today, and in this quiet place, ask yourself, *What am I meant to learn through these emotions?* Take a few moments to listen quietly for the answer to this question.

Fourth, choose an event that was significant to you today. Ask yourself, *What am I meant to learn from this event? Is there something*

*I'd like to do better next time?* With the guards of your ego down, take responsibility for your role in every interaction you had today.

Fifth, set an intention for tomorrow. This intention can be a word or a short phrase. Allow it to wash over your heart so you can remember it tomorrow.

## End-of-Day Evaluation

How am I feeling today (mood), with 10 being the best?
1  2  3  4  5  6  7  8  9  10

How am I thinking today (focus and attention), with 10 being the best?
1  2  3  4  5  6  7  8  9  10

How is my energy level today, with 10 being the best?
1  2  3  4  5  6  7  8  9  10

How did writing the thank-you note help me increase the amount of gratitude and connection I feel? How can I invite more of this spiritual energy into every day? How did completing the meditation change the way I feel about myself and others? How would continuously asking myself the questions in this meditation shift the course of my life? What was one spiritual lesson I learned from these practices today?

## Spiritual Exercise: *Life Story*

Imagine that this time in your life is the chapter in a novel. What would the chapter be called?

Take a few moments to write about yourself in the third person. As the wise, omniscient author who has all the answers to all of life's tough dilemmas, comment on the lessons "this person" was meant to learn in this chapter. Predict what joys and rewards this person has in store since you know what the future holds. Talk about the one piece of advice this "main character" needs to take right now, and how this "person" will apply it to his or her life.

## 12-Minute Meditation: *Becoming Your Ideal Self*

In this 12-minute visualization, first take time to just notice where you are today. With this new optimistic and kind lens you've cultivated, maybe you are noticing that you're just a little more peaceful, stronger, and happier than you've been in the past. Give yourself credit for that. Without any judgment, notice your thoughts and feelings. With present-minded awareness, notice the sensations that are coming to you now.

Now that you know where you are in this moment, give yourself permission to go on a brief journey somewhere else. Imagine that you're on a walk in the most beautiful place you've ever been. You can smell the flowers around you, and you hear the peaceful sounds of the ocean somewhere in the distance. A sense of euphoria and peace comes over you, and you get the sense that you're exactly where you should be at this moment.

There's a clearing up ahead, and you can see the outline of a person standing there bathed in white light. It's as if you know you're meant to meet this person. As you walk closer and closer, you realize that this person is you. It's your highest, most ideal self. As you come face to face with yourself, your two selves smile at each other.

You realize that your ideal self has something very important to tell you. It's something simple and profound, so listen very carefully. You realize that it's exactly what you were meant to hear in this moment. Hear the message not just with your ears but with your entire being. Hear it with your heart.

As you take in this profound message, you notice something happening. Visualize the part of you that has walked there and your ideal self becoming one person. In that moment, you realize that you are the same person. Your ideal self isn't outside of you. You are already good. You already have all the answers you need.

When you're ready, open your eyes. With the ideal self here with you now in the real world, see your life differently. Let it color your thoughts. Your words. And your actions.

## End-of-Day Evaluation

How am I feeling today (mood), with 10 being the best?
1 2 3 4 5 6 7 8 9 10

How am I thinking today (focus and attention), with 10 being the best?
1 2 3 4 5 6 7 8 9 10

How is my energy level today, with 10 being the best?
1 2 3 4 5 6 7 8 9 10

How did authoring my life story help me gain perspective? How would continuing to remember this shape the course of my life, goals, and actions? How can I apply the message I received from my ideal self? How can I remember that my ideal self is always here within me? What was one spiritual lesson I learned from these practices today?

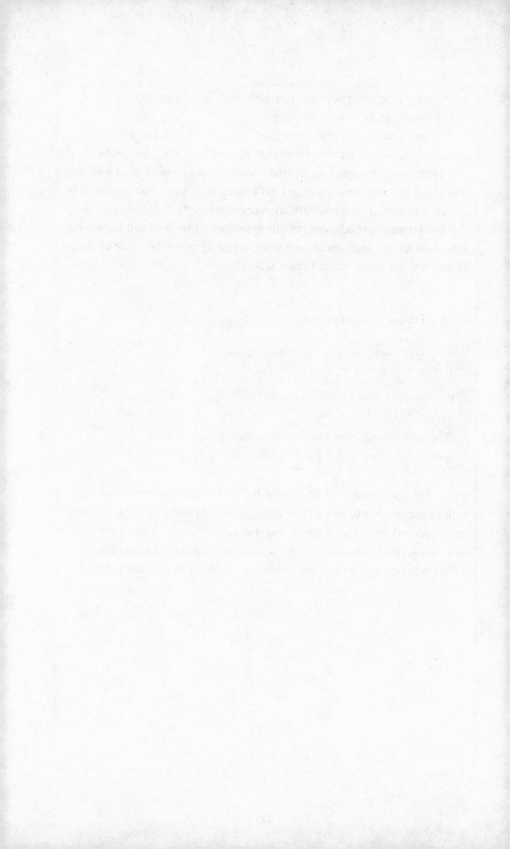

# CONCLUSION

It's my sincere hope that reading this book has changed your life in some small way. Perhaps the knowledge you have gained will change the way you talk to your spouse tonight or what you have for dinner tomorrow. Perhaps the 21-day program has helped you improve your energy. Maybe your mood has improved. Maybe you're beginning to notice your brain fog is starting to dissipate as you are struck with a sense of clarity and renewed motivation that will help you to achieve bigger goals down the road.

One of the most important lessons I hope you've learned is that you have the power to change your life. Today. Tomorrow. In the small decisions and the big ones. In your thoughts and in your deeds. In your physical health. In your psychological health. In your relationships. And in your spiritual life.

With renewed confidence, I also hope you will maintain the improvements you've made. It may not always be easy, but the rewards are well worth it. And remember: whenever you fall, you always have the opportunity to begin again. By doing so, you will be living the life you were born to live. May it be filled with purpose, clarity, and joy.

# APPENDIX A

## N-Back Tests

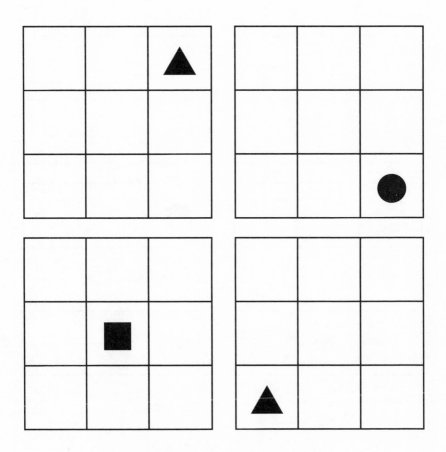

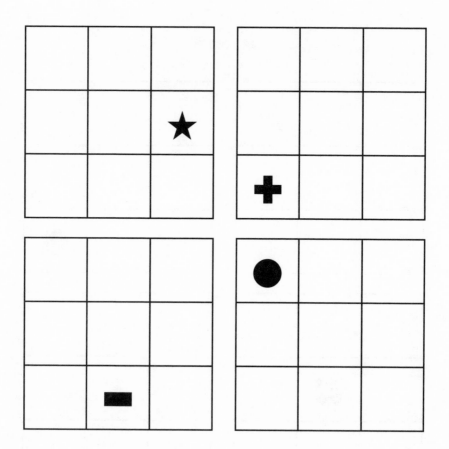

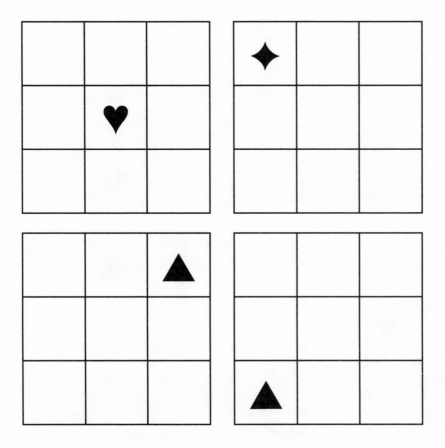

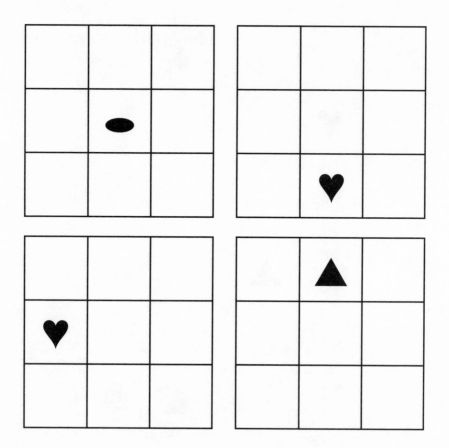

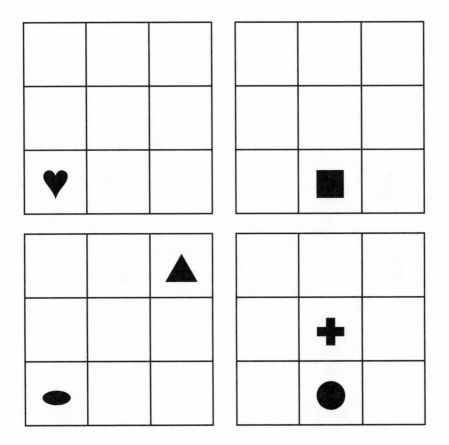

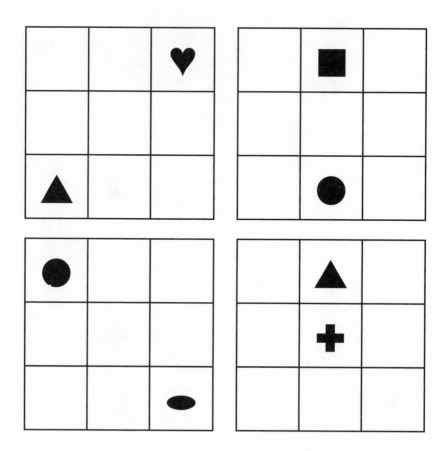

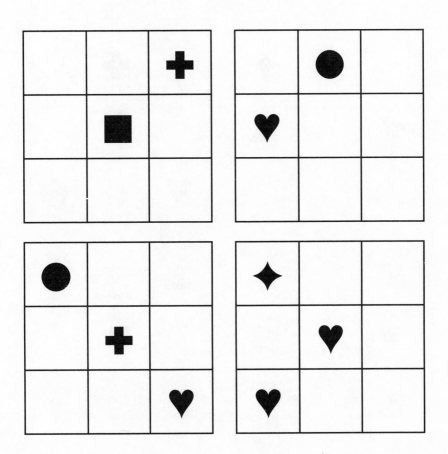

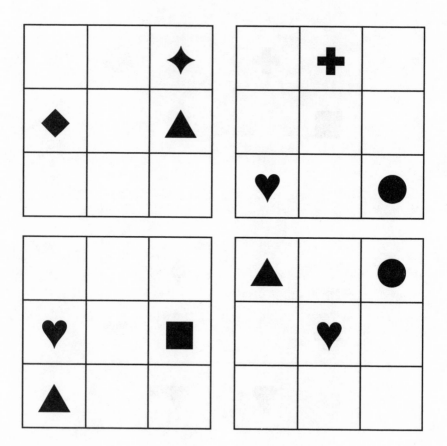

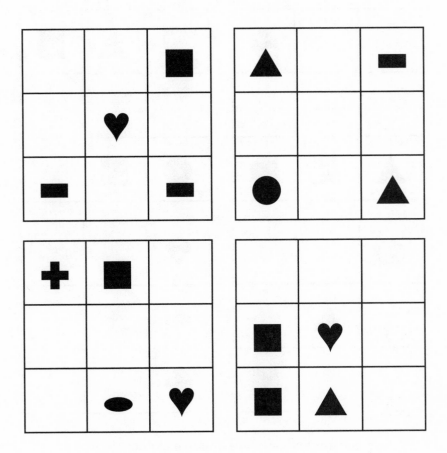

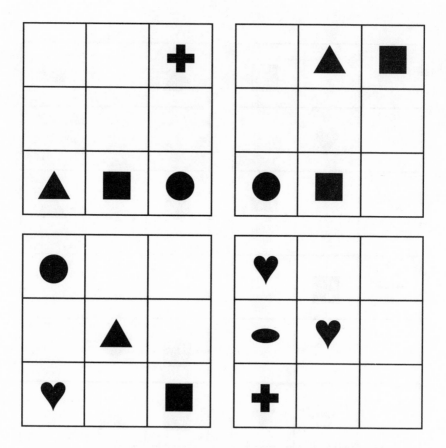

For more N-Back Tests available to print, go to
www.drmikedow.com

# APPENDIX B

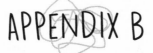

## A Blender, a Bottle, and a Buck

What's the simplest, most affordable, and most portable way to change the way you think and feel through food? Change your diet with just a blender, a bottle, and a buck. Many cheaper "green" juices are made with blood sugar–spiking apple, grape, and orange juices that can fog your brain in addition to causing weight gain. Store-bought vegetable juices can also run $5 to $10 (or more!), and most of them remove the beneficial fiber by juicing the fruits and vegetables. Blending vegetables and whole fruits with their skin on when possible means you're getting more fiber.

First, arm yourself with the best blender you can afford, like a Vitamix, Blendtec, or Ninja. I use my Vitamix Pro daily and have saved hundreds of dollars using it.

Second, get a portable bottle you can easily grab and take with you—such as a Ball wide-mouthed, one-pint canning jar or larger ones if you'd like to keep multiple servings in one jar. Having one of these handy for an afternoon snack will help you bypass chips, bread, and candy bars. I also make two to three days' worth of smoothies and juices by storing them in these bottles.

Finally, make smoothies that cost about a dollar or less per serving. One easy way to keep the costs low is to use frozen vegetables and fruits. In addition to frozen organic spinach and broccoli, you can even find frozen kale and artichokes at Trader Joe's. Of course, fresh vegetables and fruit are great, too!

By getting multiple servings of vegetables and fruits in one delicious and portable bottle, you can more easily reach your goal of having seven servings every single day—the amount that the happiest people eat every day.

These "A Blender, A Bottle, and A Buck" recipes also follow the principles outlined in *The Brain Fog Fix*.

- Keep blood-sugar spikes low by following my 80/20 rule. Try to limit the amount of fruit (not including low-sugar, fresh lemon or lime juice) in your smoothie to 20 percent or so. Keep the skin on fruits with edible skins to increase fiber to help manage blood-sugar spikes. The other 80 percent should be vegetables, lemon, lime, herbs, organic dairy, almond milk, organic soy milk, protein powder, water, and ice. Lemon, lime, fresh ginger, and fresh mint do wonders to cover up the occasionally bitter taste of vegetables.

- Favor the best type of fruit for your brain, the ones that have a low glycemic index: berries.

- Include anti-inflammatory foods and omega-3 superfoods like walnuts, ground flaxseeds, flaxseed oil, or chia seeds.

- Include anti-inflammatory vegetables and fruits with vitamins that act as cofactors that help your body produce dopamine and serotonin. They will also keep you fuller longer through the fiber they contain. Blended whole fruit and organic dairy provide a slow and steady source of carbohydrates.

- All recipes make one serving.

# WELLNESS SHOT*

1 ounce cold water
½ teaspoon ground turmeric
½ teaspoon black pepper
squeeze of lemon (optional)

*While you can just mix the ingredients in a glass, I make this shot in my blender and add fresh ginger, cayenne pepper, and ice to the ingredients.

# THE DAILY DOSE

¼ cup frozen mango (substitute: ½ pear, ½ apple, or ½ cup pineapple)
¼ cup romaine
¼ cup kale
¼ cup spinach
¼ cup broccoli
¼ cup Brussels sprouts
squeeze lemon
3 sprigs of mint
2 tablespoons chia seeds
small piece of ginger
2 cups water
½ cup ice

# BANANA NUT NO-BREAD SMOOTHIE

¼ cup walnuts
1 cup unsweetened vanilla almond milk (substitute: low-fat organic milk or unsweetened organic soy milk)
½ banana
1 cup ice
1 scoop vanilla protein powder (optional)
1 pinch cinnamon

# ABC

½ apple
½ cup beets
1 large or 20 baby carrots
small piece of ginger
½ teaspoon turmeric
pinch black pepper
1 cup water

# CHERRY VANILLA

½ cup frozen unsweetened cherries
1 cup unsweetened vanilla almond milk
1 scoop vanilla protein
½ cup ice

# CHOCOLATE-COVERED BANANA

¼ cup walnuts
1 cup unsweetened chocolate almond milk
½ banana
1 cup ice
1 scoop chocolate protein powder (optional)

# BLUEBERRY PROTEIN

½ cup frozen blueberries
½ cup kale (substitute: spinach)
1 scoop vanilla protein powder (optional)
1 cup water
1 cup ice

# THE CALIFORNIAN

¼ avocado
½ cup romaine
2 tablespoons ground flaxseeds
1 scoop vanilla protein powder
1 cup unsweetened vanilla almond milk
1 cup ice

# THE HAWAIIAN

¼ papaya
½ cup coconut water
squeeze lime
½ cup water
1 cup ice

# REFRESHER

⅓ bunch parsley
3 sprigs mint
1 cup romaine
½ large cucumber
½ apple (substitute: ½ pear)
squeeze lemon
1 cup water
1 cup ice

# POPEYE

1 cup spinach
½ banana
1 scoop vanilla protein powder
1 cup water
1 cup ice

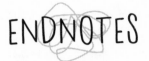
# ENDNOTES

## PART I: ALL FOGGED UP AND SCATTERED

### Chapter 1: "I Just Don't Feel Like Myself"

1.   U.S. Department of Health and Human Services, "Mental Health: A Report of the Surgeon General." Rockville, MD: National Institutes of Health, 1999.

## PART II: MOOD AND FOOD

### Chapter 3: Carbohydrates: Highs and Lows

1.   Michel Lucas et al., "Inflammatory Dietary Pattern and Risk of Depression Among Women," *Brain Behavior and Immunity* 36 (February 2014): 46–53.

2.   Brian E. Leonard, "Inflammation, Depression and Dementia: Are They Connected?" *Neurochemistry Research Journal* 32, no. 10 (October 2007): 1749–56.

3.   National Institute of Diabetes and Digestive and Kidney Diseases: Clinical Alert, "Diet and Exercise Dramatically Delay Type 2 Diabetes; Diabetes Medication Metformin Also Effective" (August 8, 2001): http://www.nlm.nih.gov/databases/alerts/diabetes01.html.

4.   T. Ohara et al., "Glucose Tolerance Status and Risk of Dementia in the Community: The Hisayama Study," *Neurology* 77, no. 12 (September 20, 2011): 1126–34.

5.   Giancarlo Logroscino, Jae Hee Kang, and Francine Grodstein, "Prospective Study of Type 2 Diabetes and Cognitive Decline in Women Aged 70–81 Years." *British Medical Journal* 328, no. 7439 (March 6, 2004): 548.

6.   Suzanne M. de la Monte and Jack Wands, "Alzheimer's Disease Is Type 3 Diabetes—Evidence Reviewed," *Journal of Diabetes Science and Technology* 2, no. 6 (November 2008): 1101–13.

7.   *Health Day,* "Lower Blood Sugar Levels May Aid Memory, Study Suggests," *US News and World Report* (October 23, 2013): http://health.usnews.com/health-news/news/articles/2013/10/23/lower-blood-sugar-levels-may-aid-memory-study-suggests.

8.   Moyra E. Mortby et al., "High 'Normal' Blood Glucose Is Associated with Decreased Brain Volume and Cognitive Performance in the 60s: The PATH through Life Study," *Public Library of Science* 8, no. 9 (September 4, 2013):

http://www.plosone.org/article/info%3Adoi%2F10.1371%2Fjournal.
pone.0073697.

9.  Paul K. Crane et al., "Glucose Levels and Risk of Dementia," *New England Journal of Medicine* 369 (August 8, 2013): 540–48.

10. James Salisi, "Hypertension and Dementia: Is There a Link?" MIMS Phillipines (April 2014): http://pub.mims.com/Philippines/topic/Medical-Tribune-PH/Hypertension-and-dementia-is-there-a-link?_s1=5H1vYZCNblvxgSfg_K7Tacwwe7U1.

11. Alzheimer's Disease International Policy Brief, "The Global Impact of Dementia 2013–2050," Alzheimer's Disease International (December 2013): http://www.alz.co.uk/research/G8-policy-brief.

12. Ewan C. McKay, Thomas M. Fries, and Paul E. Gold, "Decreases in Rat Extracellular Hippocampal Glucose Concentration Associated with Cognitive Demand During a Spatial Task," *Proceedings of the National Academy of Sciences of the United States of America* 97, no. 6 (March 14, 2000): 2881–85.

13. Randall J. Kaplan et al., "Cognitive Performance Is Associated with Glucose Regulation in Healthy Elderly Persons and Can Be Enhanced with Glucose and Dietary Carbohydrates," *American Journal Clinical Nutrition* 72, no. 3 (September 2000): 825–36.

14. Young-In Kwon, Emmanouil Apostolidis, and Kalidas Shetty, "Inhibitory Potential of Wine and Tea Against A-Amylase and A-Glucosidase for Management of Hyperglycemia Linked to Type 2 Diabetes," *Journal of Food Biochemistry* 32, no. 1 (February 2008): 15–31.

15. Ibid.

## Chapter 4: Dietary Fats: The Good, the Bad, and the Ugly

1.  Rosebud O. Roberts et al., "Relative Intake of Macronutrients Impacts Risk of Mild Cognitive Impairment or Dementia," *Journal of Alzheimer's Disease* 32, no. 2 (2012): 329–39.

2.  Q. Li et al., "Docosahexaenoic Acid Changes Lipid Composition and Interleukin-2 Receptor Signaling in Membrane Rafts," *The Journal of Lipid Research* 46 (2005): 1904–13.

3.  Goodarz Danaei et al., "The Preventable Causes of Death in the United States: Comparative Risk Assessment of Dietary, Lifestyle, and Metabolic Risk Factors," *PLOS Medicine* 6, no. 4 (April 28, 2009): http://www.plosmedicine.org/article/info%3Adoi%2F10.1371%2Fjournal.pmed.1000058.

4.  L. S. Rallidis et al., "Dietary Alpha-Linolenic Acid Decreases C-Reactive Protein, Serum Amyloid A and Interleukin-6 in Dyslipidaemic Patients," *Atherosclerosis* 167, no. 2 (April 2003): 237–42.

Endnotes

5. Ernst J. Schaefer et al., "Plasma Phosphatidylcholine Docosahexaenoic Acid Content and Risk of Dementia and Alzheimer Disease: the Framingham Heart Study," *JAMA* 63, no. 11 (November 2006): 1545–50.

6. Rhian Edwards et al., "Omega-3 Polyunsaturated Fatty Acid Levels in the Diet and in Red Blood Cell Membranes of Depressed Patients," *Journal of Affective Disorders* 48, nos. 2–3 (March 1, 1998): 149–55; L. J. Stevens et al., "Essential Fatty Acid Metabolism in Boys with Attention-Deficit Hyperactivity Disorder," *American Journal of Clinical Nutrition* 62 (1995): 761–68.

7. Karen M. Silvers and Kate M. Scott, "Fish Consumption and Self-Reported Physical and Mental Health Status," *Public Health Nutrition* 5 (June 2002): 427–31.

8. M. B. Raeder et al., "Associations between Cod Liver Oil Use and Symptoms of Depression: The Hordaland Study," *Journal of Affective Disorders* 101 (August 2007): 245–49.

9. F. Lespérance et al., "The Efficacy of Omega-3 Supplementation for Major Depression: A Randomized Controlled Trial," *Journal of Clinical Psychiatry* 72, no. 8 (August 2011): 1054–62; Janice K. Kiecolt-Glaser et al., "Omega-3 Supplementation Lowers Inflammation and Anxiety in Medical Students: A Randomized Controlled Trial," *Brain Behavior and Immunity* 25, no. 8 (November 2011): 1725–34.

10. Boukje Maria van Gelder, Marja Tijhuis, and Daan Kalmijn, "Fish Consumption, N-3 Fatty Acids, and Subsequent 5-y Cognitive Decline in Elderly Men: the Zutphen Elderly Study," *American Journal of Clinical Nutrition* 85, no. 4 (April 2007): 1142–47; Greg M. Cole and Sally A. Frautschy, "Docosahexaenoic Acid Protects from Amyloid and Dendritic Pathology in an Alzheimer's Disease Mouse Model," *Nutrition and Health* 18, no. 3 (2006): 249–59.

11. David Benton, "Selenium Intake, Mood and Other Aspects of Psychological Functioning," *Nutritional Neuroscience* 5, no. 6 (December 2002): 363–74; N. Mokhber et al., "Effect of Supplementation with Selenium on Postpartum Depression: A Randomized Double-Blind Placebo-Controlled Trial," *Journal of Maternal-Fetal and Neonatal Medicine* 24, no. 1 (January 2011): 104–08.

12. Claudine Berr, Josiane Arnaud, and Tasnime N. Akbaraly, "Selenium and Cognitive Impairment: A Brief-Review Based on Results from the EVA Study," *Biofactors* 32, no. 2 (March 2012): 139–44.

13. K. L. Weaver et al., "The Content of Favorable and Unfavorable Polyunsaturated Fatty Acids Found in Commonly Eaten Fish," *Journal of the American Dietary Association* 108, no. 7 (July 2008): 1178–85.

14. Damian P. Wojcik et al., "Mercury Toxicity Presenting as Chronic Fatigue, Memory Impairment and Depression: Diagnosis, Treatment, Susceptibility, and Outcomes in a New Zealand General Practice Setting (1994–2006)," *Neuroendocrinology Letters* 27, no. 4 (August 2006): 415–23.

15. Gary J. Myers and Philip W. Davidson, "Does Methylmercury Have a Role in Causing Developmental Disabilities in Children?" *Environmental Health Perspectives* 108, Supplement 3 (June 2000): 413–20.

16. E. Oken et al., "Maternal Fish Consumption, Hair Mercury, and Infant Cognition in a U.S. Cohort," *Environmental Health Perspectives* 113, no. 10 (October 2005): 1376–80.

17. Dariush Mozaffarian and Eric B. Rimm, "Fish Intake, Contaminants, and Human Health: Evaluating the Risks and the Benefits," *JAMA* 297, no. 6 (February 14, 2007): 590.

18. Ousséni Ouédraogo and Marc Amyot, "Effects of Various Cooking Methods and Food Components on Bioaccessibility of Mercury from Fish," *Environmental Research* 111, no. 8 (November 2011): 1064–69.

19. Paul H. A. Steegmans et al., "Higher Prevalence of Depressive Symptoms in Middle-Aged Men with Low Serum Cholesterol Levels," *Psychosomatic Medicine* 62, no. 2 (March–April 2000): 205–11; Myriam Horsten et al., "Depressive Symptoms, Social Support, and Lipid Profile in Healthy Middle-Aged Women," *Psychosomatic Medicine* 59, no. 5 (May–June 1998): 521–28.

20. Claudine Berr et al., "Olive Oil and Cognition: Results from the Three-City Study," *Dementia and Geriatric Cognitive Disorders* 28, no. 4 (October 2009): 357–64.

21. C. Samieri et al., "Olive Oil Consumption, Plasma Oleic Acid, and Stroke Incidence: The Three-City Study," *Neurology* (June 2011): http://www.neurology. org/content/early/2011/06/15/WNL.0b013e318220abeb.abstract.

22. Nikolaos Scarmeas et al., "Mediterranean Diet and Mild Cognitive Impairment," *Archives of Neurology* 66, no. 2 (February 2009): 216–25.

23. Almudena Sánchez-Villegas et al., "Association of the Mediterranean Dietary Pattern with the Incidence of Depression: The Seguimiento Universidad de Navarra/University of Navarra Follow-up (SUN) Cohort," *MPH Archives of General Psychiatry* 66, no. 10 (October 2009): 1090–98.

24. Almudena Sánchez-Villegas et al., "Dietary Fat Intake and the Risk of Depression: The SUN Project," *PLOS One* (January 26, 2011): http://www.plosone.org/article/ info%3Adoi%2F10.1371%2Fjournal.pone.0016268.

## Chapter 5: Proteins: The Building Blocks of the Body—and the Brain

1. W. N. Jefferson et al., "Adverse Effects on Female Development and Reproduction in CD-1 Mice Following Neonatal Exposure to the Phytoestrogen Genistein at Environmentally Relevant Doses," *Biology of Reproduction* 73 no. 4 (October 1, 2005): 798–806.

2.  Y. Toyohira et al., "Stimulatory Effects of the Soy Phytoestrogen Genistein on Noradrenaline Transporter and Serotonin Transporter Activity," *Molecular Nutrition and Food Research* 54, no. 4 (April 2010): 516–24; Maria Luisa Casini et al., "Psychological Assessment of the Effects of Treatment with Phytoestrogens on Postmenopausal Women: A Randomized, Double-Blind, Crossover, Placebo-Controlled Study," *Fertility and Sterility* 85, no. 4 (April 2006): 972–78.

3.  J. Hellhammer et al., "Effects of Soy Lecithin Phosphatidic Acid and Phosphatidylserine Complex (PAS) on the Endocrine and Psychological Responses to Mental Stress," *Stress* 7, no. 2 (June 2004): 119–26.

4.  Liqin Zhao and Roberta Diaz Brinton, "WHI and WHIMS Follow-up and Human Studies of Soy Isoflavones on Cognition," *Expert Review of Neurotherapeutics* 7, no. 11 (November 2007):1549–64.

5.  Cynthia A. Daley et al., "A Review of Fatty Acid Profiles and Antioxidant Content in Grass-Fed and Grain-Fed Beef," *Nutrition Journal* 2010 (March 2010): http://www.nutritionj.com/content/9/1/10.

6.  P. I. Ponte et al., "Restricting the Intake of a Cereal-Based Feed in Free-Range-Pastured Poultry: Effects on Performance and Meat Quality," *Poultry Science* 87, no. 10 (October 2008): 2032–42; P. I. Ponte et al., "Influence of Pasture Intake on the Fatty Acid Composition, and Cholesterol, Tocopherols, and Tocotrienols Content in Meat from Free-Range Broilers," *Poultry Science* 87, no. 1 (January 2008): 80–88; Angela Gabriella D'Alessandro et al., "How the Nutritional Value and Consumer Acceptability of Suckling Lambs Meat Is Affected by the Maternal Feeding System," *Small Ruminant Research* 106, no. 2 (February 2012) 83–91.

7.  Mozaffarian and Rimm, "Fish Intake, Contaminants, and Human Health: Evaluating the Risks and the Benefits."

8.  International Agency for Research on Cancer, "IARC Monographs on the Evaluation of the Carcinogenic Risk of Chemicals to Humans," 32 (1983); M. Gerhardsson de Verdier et al., "Meat, Cooking Methods and Colorectal Cancer: A Case-Referent Study in Stockholm," *International Journal of Cancer* 49, no. 4 (October 21, 1991): 520–25.

9.  Rebecca J. Scharf, Ryan Demmer, and Mark DeBoer, "Longitudinal Evaluation of Milk Type Consumed and Weight Status in Preschoolers," *Archives of Disease in Childhood* 98 (March 2013): 335–40.

10. Liesbeth A. Smit et al., "Conjugated Linoleic Acid in Adipose Tissue and Risk of Myocardial Infarction," *American Journal of Clinical Nutrition* 92, no 1 (July 2010): 34–40.

11. Jeff Mulhollem, "Research Shows Eggs from Pastured Chickens May Be More Nutritious," *Penn State News* (July 10, 2010): http://news.psu.edu/story/166143/2010/07/20/research-shows-eggs-pastured-chickens-may-be-more-nutritious.

12. Marianne J. Engelhart et al., "Dietary Intake of Antioxidants and Risk of Alzheimer Disease," *Journal of the American Medical Association* 287 (June 26, 2002): 3223–29; Anthony E. Lang and Andres M. Lozano, "Parkinson's Disease. First of Two Parts," *New England Journal of Medicine* 339 (October 8, 1998): 111–14.

## Chapter 6: A Modified Mediterranean Diet

1.  David G. Blanchflower et al., "Is Psychological Well-Being Linked to the Consumption of Fruit and Vegetables?" *Social Indicators Research* 114, no. 3 (December 2013): 785–801.

2.  Undurti N. Das, "Folic Acid and Polyunsaturated Fatty Acids Improve Cognitive Function and Prevent Depression, Dementia, and Alzheimer's Disease—But How and Why?" *Prostaglandins, Leukotrienes and Essential Fatty Acids* 78, no. 1 (January 2008): 11–19.

3.  Henry Silver, "Vitamin B12 Levels Are Low in Hospitalized Psychiatric Patients," *Israel Journal of Psychiatry and Related Sciences* 37, no. 1 (2000): 41–45.

4.  Adit A. Ginde et al., "Demographic Differences and Trends of Vitamin D Insufficiency in the US Population, 1988–2004," *Archives of Internal Medicine* 169, no. 6 (2009): 626–32.

5.  Rebecca E. S. Anglin et al., "Vitamin D Deficiency and Depression in Adults: Systematic Review and Meta-Analysis," *The British Journal of Psychiatry* 202 (2013): 100–7.

6.  S. M. Seifert et al., "Health Effects of Energy Drinks on Children, Adolescents, and Young Adults," *Pediatrics* 127, no. 3 (March 2011): 511–28.

7.  Michelle Castello, "Sweetened Drinks Linked to Depression in Older Adults," *CBS News* (January 10, 2013): www.cbsnews.com/news/sweetened-drinks-linked-to-depression-in-older-adults/.

8.  Honor Whiteman, "Four Cups of Coffee a Day Linked to Early Death," *Medical News Today* (August 16, 2013): www.medicalnewstoday.com/articles/264778.php.

9.  Marjo H. Eskelinen et al., "Midlife Coffee and Tea Drinking and the Risk of Late-Life Dementia: A Population-Based CAIDE Study," *Journal of Alzheimer's Disease* 16, no. 1 (2009): 85–91.

10. Edward J. Neafsey and Michael A Collins, "Moderate Alcohol Consumption and Cognitive Risk," *Neuropsychiatric Disease and Treatment* 7 (2011): 465–84.

11. A. Imhof et al., "Overall Alcohol Intake, Beer, Wine, and Systemic Markers of Inflammation in Western Europe: Results from Three MONICA Samples (Augsburg, Glasgow, Lille)," *European Heart Journal* 25, no. 23 (December 2004): 2092–2100.

12. John A. Ringman et al., "A Potential Role of the Curry Spice Curcumin in Alzheimer's Disease," *Current Alzheimer's Research* 2, no. 2 (April 2005): 131–36.

## PART III: THE GUNK THAT CLOGS UP YOUR BRAIN

### Chapter 7: Too Many Meds

1. Centers for Disease Control and Prevention, "Emergency Department Visits Involving Nonmedical Use of Selected Prescription Drugs, United States, 2004–2008," *Morbidity and Mortality Weekly Report* 59, no. 23 (June 18, 2010): 705–9.

2. Malcolm H. Lader, M. Ron, and H. Petursson, "Computed Axial Brain Tomography in Long-Term Benzodiazepine Users," *Psychological Medicine* 14 (1984): 203–6.

3. Rajaa Lagnaoui et al., "Benzodiazepine Use and Risk of Dementia: A Nested Case-Control Study," *Journal of Clinical Epidemiology* 55, no. 3 (March 2002): 314–18.

4. P. R. Tata et al., "Lack of Cognitive Recovery Following Withdrawal from Long-Term Benzodiazepine Use," *Psychological Medicine* 24, no. 1 (1994): 203–13.

5. Melinda J. Barker et al., "Cognitive Effects of Long-Term Benzodiazepine Use: A Meta-Analysis," *CNS Drugs* 18, no. 1 (2004): 37–48.

6. R. Bruce Lydiard et al., "Emergence of Depressive Symptoms in Patients Receiving Alprazolam for Panic Disorder," *The American Journal of Psychiatry* 144, no. 5 (May 1987): 664–65.

7. E. Schweizer and K. Rickels, "Benzodiazepine Dependence and Withdrawal: A Review of the Syndrome and Its Clinical Management," *Acta Psychaitrica Scandinavica* 393 (1998): 95–101.

8. Isaac M. Marks et al., "The 'Efficacy' of Alprazolam in Panic Disorder and Agoraphobia: A Critique of Recent Reports," *Archives of General Psychiatry* 46, no. 7 (July 1989): 668–70.

9. World Health Organization, "The Global Burden of Disease: 2004 Update, Table A2: Burden of Disease in DALYs by Cause, Sex and Income Group in WHO Regions, Estimates for 2004," (Geneva, Switzerland: World Health Organization, 2008): 36.

10. John S. March et al., "The Treatment of Adolescents with Depression Study (TADS), Long Term Effectiveness and Safety Outcomes," *Archives of General Psychiatry* 64, no. 10 (October 2007): 1132–43.

11. H. M. Gonzalez et al., "Depression Care in the United States: Too Little for Too Few," *Archives of General Psychiatry* 67, no. 1 (January 2010): 37–46.

12. A. L. Montejo et al., "Incidence of Sexual Dysfunction Associated with Antidepressant Agents: A Prospective Multicenter Study of 1022 Outpatients.

Spanish Working Group for the Study of Psychotropic-Related Sexual Dysfunction," *The Journal of Clinical Psychiatry* 62, Supplement 3 (2002): 10–21.

13. Robert P. Vertes and Kathleen E. Eastman, "The Case Against Memory Consolidation in REM Sleep," *Behavioral and Brain Sciences* 23, no. 6 (2000): 867–76.

14. Jerome M. Siegel and Michael A. Rogawski, "A Function for REM sleep: Regulation of Noradrenergic Receptor Sensitivity," *Brain Research Review* 13 (1988): 213.

15. Robert J. Valuck, Heather D. Orton, and Anne M. Libby, "Antidepressant Discontinuation and Risk of Suicide Attempt," *The Journal of Clinical Psychiatry* 70, no. 8 (2009): 1069–77.

16. Lisa Cosgrove et al., "Antidepressants and Breast and Ovarian Cancer Risk: A Review of the Literature and Researchers' Financial Associations with Industry," *PLOS One* (April 6, 2011): http://www.plosone.org/article/info%3Adoi%2F10.1371%2Fjournal.pone.0018210.

17. C. M. Kelly et al., "Selective Serotonin Reuptake Inhibitors and Breast Cancer Mortality in Women Receiving Tamoxifen: A Population Based Cohort Study," *British Medical Journal* 2010 (February 8, 2010): 340.

18. J. W. Smoller et al., "Antidepressant Use and Risk of Incident Cardiovascular Morbidity and Mortality Among Postmenopausal Women in the Women's Health Initiative Study," *Archives of Internal Medicine* 169, no. 22 (2009): 2128–39.

19. Jordan W. Turner et al., "Selective Publication of Antidepressant Trials and Its Influence on Apparent Efficacy," *New England Journal of Medicine* 358 (2007): 252–60.

20. Irving Kirsch, *The Emperor's New Drugs: Exploding the Antidepressant Myth* (New York: Basic Books, 2010): 28.

21. Shima Jazayeri et al., "Comparison of Therapeutic Effects of Omega-3 Fatty Acid Eicosapentaenoic Acid and Fluoxetine, Separately and in Combination, in Major Depressive Disorder," *Australian and New Zealand Journal of Psychiatry* 42, no. 3 (2008): 192–98.

22. Mark Hamer et al., "Anti-depressant Medication Use and C-Reactive Protein: Results from Two Population-Based Studies," *Brain Behavior and Immunity* 25, no. 1 (January 2011): 168–73; Jennifer L. Warner-Schmidt et al., "Antidepressant Effects of Selective Serotonin Reuptake Inhibitors (SSRIs) Are Attenuated by Antiinflammatory Drugs in Mice and Humans," *Proceedings of the National Academy of Sciences* 108, no. 22 (May 31, 2011): 9262–67.

23. Rajeev Krishnadas and Jonathan Cavanagh, "Depression: An Inflammatory Illness?" *Journal of Neurology, Neurosurgery, and Psychiatry* 83 (2012): 495–502.

24. Marie Kim Wium-Andersen et al., "Elevated C-Reactive Protein Levels, Psychological Distress, and Depression in 73,131 Individuals," *Journal of the American Medical Association Psychiatry* 70, no. 2 (2013): 176–84.

25. R. Dantzer et al., "From Inflammation to Sickness and Depression: When the Immune System Subjugates the Brain," *Nature Reviews Neuroscience* 9, no. 1 (January 2008): 46–56.

26. Stephen V. Faraone et al., "What Is the Prevalence of Adult ADHD? Results of a Population Screen of 966 Adults," *Journal of Attention Disorders* 9, no. 2 (2005): 384–91.

27. H. Hart et al., "Meta-analysis of Functional Magnetic Resonance Imaging Studies of Inhibition and Attention in Attention-deficit/Hyperactivity Disorder Exploring Task-Specific, Stimulant Medication, and Age Effects," *Journal of the American Medical Association Psychiatry* 70, no. 2 (2013): 185–98.

28. Alan Schwarz, "Drowned in a Sea of Prescriptions," *The New York Times* (February 2, 2013): http://www.nytimes.com/2013/02/03/us/concerns-about-adhd-practices-and-amphetamine-addiction.html.

29. S. J. Shoptaw et al., "Treatment for Amphetamine Withdrawal," *Cochrane Database of Systemic Reviews* 2 (April 15, 2009): CD003021.

30. Myriam Sollman et al., "Detection of Feigned ADHD in College Students," *Psychological Assessment* 22, no. 2 (June 2010): 325–35.

31. Sean Esteban McCabe et al., "Non-Medical Use of Prescription Stimulants Among US College Students: Prevalence and Correlates from a National Survey," *Addiction* 99 (2005): 96–106.

32. IMS Institute for Healthcare Informatics, "The Use of Medicines in the United States: Review of 2011," 42 (April 2012): https://www.imshealth.com/ims/Global/Content/Insights/IMS%20Institute%20for%20Healthcare%20Informatics/IHII_Medicines_in_U.S_Report_2011.pdf.

33. A. L. Culver et al., "Statin Use and Risk of Diabetes Mellitus in Postmenopausal Women in the Women's Health Initiative," *Archives of Internal Medicine* 172, no. 2 (2012): 144–52.

34. Ross Pelton et al., *Drug-Induced Nutrient Depletion Handbook* (Hudson, OH: Lexi-Comp, 2001).

35. Zeyan Liew et al., "Acetaminophen Use During Pregnancy, Behavioral Problems, and Hyperkinetic Disorders," *Journal of the Academy of the American Medical Association Pediatrics* 168, no. 4 (February 24, 2014): 313–20.

36. Randall Espinoza and Jürgen Unützer, "Diagnosis and Management of Late-life Depression," *UpToDate* (2013): http://www.uptodate.com/contents/diagnosis-and-management-of-late-life-depression#h1.

## Chapter 8: Taking on Toxins

1. Philippe Grandjean and Philip Landrigan, "Neurobehavioural effects of developmental toxicity," *The Lancet Neurology* 13, no. 3 (March 2014): 330–38.

2. "Manganese in Drinking Water: Study Suggests Adverse Effects on Children's Intellectual Abilities," Phys.org (September 20, 2010): http://phys.org/news204177632.html.

3. Benjamin J. Apelberg et al., "Cord Serum Concentrations of Perfluorooctane Sulfonate (PFOS) and Perfluorooctanoate (PFOA) in Relation to Weight and Size at Birth," *Environmental Health Perspectives* 115, no. 11 (November 2007): 1670–76.

4. Vaughn Barry, Andrea Winquist, and Kyle Steenland, "Perfluorooctanoic Acid (PFOA) Exposures and Incident Cancers Among Adults Living Near a Chemical Plant," *Environmental Health Perspectives* 121, no. 11–12 (November–December 2013): http://ehp.niehs.nih.gov/1306615/.

5. Haiyan Tong et al., "Omega-3 Fatty Acid Supplementation Appears to Attenuate Particulate Air Pollution-induced Cardiac Effects and Lipid Changes in Healthy Middle-aged Adults," *Environmental Health Perspectives* 120, no. 7 (2012): 952.

## PART IV: LIFESTYLE READJUSTMENTS

## Chapter 9: Our Way Too Sedentary Lives

1. Brad Plumer, "Commuting in the US is Long and Hellish—But At Least It Isn't Getting Worse," *The Washington Post* (March 5, 2013): http://www.washingtonpost.com/blogs/wonkblog/wp/2013/03/05/commuting-in-the-u-s-is-long-and-hellish-but-at-least-it-hasnt-gotten-worse/.

2. R. C. Brownson et al., "Declining Rates of Physical Activity in the United States: What Are the Contributors?" *Annual Review of Public Health* 26 (2005):421–43.

3. Nielsen Company, Three Screen Report, Q1 2010: http://www.nielsen.com/us/en/insights/news/2010/what-consumers-watch-nielsens-q1-2010-three-screen-report.html.

4. Nielsen Company, TV usage trends: Q3 and Q4 2010: http://www.nielsen.com/content/dam/corporate/us/en/newswire/uploads/2011/03/State-of-the-Media-TV-Q3-Q4-2010.pdf.

5. Anders Grøntved and Frank B. Hu, "Television Viewing and Risk of Type 2 Diabetes, Cardiovascular Disease, and All-Cause Mortality," *JAMA* 305, no. 23 (June 15, 2011): 2448–55.

6. P. C. Hallal et al., "Global Physical Activity Levels: Surveillance Prospects, Pitfalls, and Progress," *The Lancet* 380, no. 9838 (July 2012): 247–57.

7. *Health Day* "Too Much Sitting After 60 May Lead to Disability, Study Says," UC San Diego Health System (February 19, 2014): http://myhealth.ucsd.edu/ YourFamily/Men/NewsRecent/6,685016#sthash.hpews3JH.dpuf.

8. Bonnie Berkowitz and Patterson Clark, "The Health Hazards of Sitting," *Washington Post* (January 20, 2014): http://apps.washingtonpost.com/g/page/ national/the-health-hazards-of-sitting/750/.

9. David W. Dunstan et al., "Breaking Up Prolonged Sitting Reduces Postprandial Glucose and Insulin Responses Diabetes Care," *Diabetes Care* (May 2012): 976–83.

10. Tatiana Y. Warren et al., "Sedentary Behaviors Increase Risk of Cardiovascular Disease Mortality in Men," *Medicine and Science in Sports and Exercise* 42, no. 5 (May 2010): 879–85.

11. Michael Babyak et al., "Exercise Treatment for Major Depression: Maintenance of Therapeutic Benefit at 10 Months," *Psychosomatic Medicine* 62, no. 5 (September–October 2000): 633–38.

12. K. I. Erickson et al., "Physical Activity Predicts Gray Matter Volume in Late Adulthood: The Cardiovascular Health Study," *Neurology* 75, no. 16 (October 13, 2010): 1415–22.

13. Robert D. Abbott et al., "Walking and Dementia in Physically Capable Elderly Men," *Journal of the American Medical Association* 292, no. 12 (September 22, 2004): 1447–53.

14. Joanna R. Erion et al., "Obesity Elicits Interleukin 1-mediated Deficits in Hippocampal Synaptic Plasticity," *Journal of Neuroscience* 34, no. 7 (February 12, 2014): 2618–31.

15. Robert E. England, David R. Morgan, and John E. Pelissero, *Managing Urban America* (Thousand Oaks, CA: CQ Press, 2011).

16. Christine M. Hoehner et al., "Commuting Distance, Cardiorespiratory Fitness, and Metabolic Risk," *American Journal of Preventive Medicine* 42, no. 6 (June 2012): 571–78.

## Chapter 10: Light, Sleep, and Technology

1. Carla S. Möller-Levet et al., "Effects of Insufficient Sleep on Circadian Rhythmicity and Expression Amplitude of the Human Blood Transcriptome," *Proceedings of the National Academy of Sciences of the United States of America* 110, no. 12 (2013): http://www.pnas.org/content/110/12/E1132.abstract.

2. Helen C. Thorne et al., "Daily and Seasonal Variation in the Spectral Composition of Light Exposure in Humans," *Chronobiology International* 26 (2009): 854–66.

3. Drew Dawson and Kathryn Reid, "Fatigue, Alcohol and Performance Impairment," *Nature* 388 (July 17, 1997): 235.

4. Hans P. A. Van Dongen et al., "The Cumulative Cost of Additional Wakefulness: Dose-Response Effects on Neurobehavioral Functions and Sleep Physiology from Chronic Sleep Restriction and Total Sleep Deprivation," *Sleep* 26, no. 2 (2003): 117–26.

5. Jason Varughese and Richard P. Allen, "Fatal Accidents Following Changes in Daylight Savings Time: The American Experience," *Sleep Medicine* 2, no. 1 (2001): 31–36.

6. Rupert Lanzenberger et al., "Cortisol Plasma Levels in Social Anxiety Disorder Patients Correlate with Serotonin-1A Receptor Binding in Limbic Brain Regions," *The International Journal of Neuropsychopharmacology* 13, no. 9 (2010): 1129–43.

7. Lulu Xie et al., "Sleep Drives Metabolite Clearance from the Adult Brain," *Science* 342, no. 6156 (October 18, 2013): 373–77.

8. Jae-Eun Kang et al., "Amyloid-Aβ Dynamics Are Regulated by Orexin and the Sleep-Wake Cycle," *Science* 326, no. 5955 (November 13, 2009): 1005–7.

9. Michele Bellesi et al., "Effects of Sleep and Wake on Oligodendrocytes and Their Precursors," *The Journal of Neuroscience* 33, no. 36 (September 4, 2013): 14288–300.

10. Kathryn J. Reid et al., "Timing and Intensity of Light Correlate with Body Weight in Adults," *PLOS One* (April 2, 2014): http://www.plosone.org/article/info%3Adoi%2F10.1371%2Fjournal.pone.0092251.

11. Thomas C. Erren, Russel J. Reiter, and Claus Piekarski, "Light, Timing of Biological Rhythms, and Chronodisruption in Man," *Naturwissenschaften* 90 (2003): 485–94.

12. Anthony Miller and Leslie Gaudette, "Breast Cancer in Circumpolar Inuit, 1969–1988," *Acta Oncologica* 35 (1996): 577–80; Orrenzo B. Snyder, Janet J. Kelly, and Anne P. Lanier, "Prostate Cancer in Alaskan Native Men, 1969–2003," *International Journal of Circumpolar Health* 65 (2006): 8–17.

13. Michael Karasek et al., "Serum Melatonin Circadian Profiles in Women Suffering from Cervical Cancer," *Journal of Pineal Research* 39 (2005): 73–76.

14. Francesco P. Cappuccio et al., "Sleep Duration and All-Cause Mortality: A Systematic Review and Meta-Analysis of Prospective Studies," *Sleep* 33, no. 5 (May 1, 2010): 585–92.

15. Harvey R. Colten and Bruce M. Altevogt, ed., *Sleep Disorders and Sleep Deprivation: An Unmet Public Health Problem* (Washington, DC: National Academies Press, 2006): 1.

16. Stephanie Saul, "Record Sales of Sleeping Pills are Causing Worries," *New York Times* (February 7, 2006): http://www.nytimes.com/2006/02/07/business/07sleep.html.

17. IMS Institute for Healthcare Informatics, "The Use of Medicines in the United States: Review of 2011," 42 (April 2012).

18. Saul, "Record Sales of Sleeping Pills are Causing Worries."

19. Heath Gilmore, "Sleeping Pill Safety under Federal Review," *Sydney Morning Herald* (March 11, 2007): http://www.smh.com.au/news/national/sleeping-pill-safety-under-federal-review/2007/03/10/1173478729115.html.

20. "Kennedy's Crash Highlights Dangers of Ambien," *ABC News* (May 5, 2006): http://abcnews.go.com/Health/story?id=1927026.

21. L. Reidy et al., "The Incidence of Zolpidem Use in Suspected DUI Drivers in Miami-Dade Florida: A Comparative Study Using Immunalysis Zolpidem ELISA KIT and Gas Chromatography-Mass Spectrometry Screening," *Journal of Analytic Toxicology* 32, no. 8 (2008): 688–94.

22. Food and Drug Administration, "FDA Requires Lower Dosing of Zolpidem," *The Medical Letter on Drugs and Therapeutics* 55, no. 1408 (January 21, 2013): 5; Food and Drug Administration, "Risk of Next-Morning Impairment After Use of Insomnia Drugs; FDA Requires Lower Recommended Doses for Certain Drugs Containing Zolpidem (Ambien, Ambien CR, Edluar, and Zolpimist)," *FDA Drug Safety Commission* (January 10, 2013): http://www.fda.gov/downloads/Drugs/DrugSafety/UCM335007.pdf.

23. Jennifer Glass et al., "Sedative Hypnotics in Older People with Insomnia: Meta-Analysis of Risks and Benefits," *British Medical Journal* 335 (November 17, 2005): 1169.

24. Substance Abuse and Mental Health Services Administration, "Emergency Department Visits for Adverse Reactions Involving the Medication Zolpidem," *The Dawn Report* (May 1, 2013): http://archive.samhsa.gov/data/2k13/DAWN079/sr079-Zolpidem.htm.

25. Daniel F. Kripke, Robert D. Langer, and Lawrence E. Kline, "Hypnotics' Association with Mortality or Cancer: A Matched Cohort Study," *British Medical Journal Open* (February 7, 2012): http://bmjopen.bmj.com/content/2/1/e000850.full.

26. Ian Parker, "The Big Sleep," *The New Yorker* (December 9, 2013): http://www.newyorker.com/magazine/2013/12/09/the-big-sleep-2.

27. Jui-HsiuTsai et al., "Zolpidem-Induced Amnesia and Somnambulism: Rare Occurrences?" *European Neuropsychopharmacology* 19, no. 1 (January 2009): 74–76.

28. P. Kintz, "Bioanalytical Procedures for Detection of Chemical Agents in Hair in the Case of Drug-Facilitated Crimes," *Analytical and Bioanalytical Chemistry* 388 no. 7 (August 2007): 1467–74.

29. Constantin R. Soldatos, Dimitris G. Dikeos, and Anne Whitehead, "Tolerance and Rebound Insomnia with Rapidly Eliminated Hypnotics: A Meta-analysis of Sleep Laboratory Studies," *International Clinical Psychopharmacology* 14, no. 5 (September 1999): 287–303.

30. M. T. Smith et al., "Comparative Meta-Analysis of Pharmacotherapy and Behavior Therapy for Persistent Insomnia," *American Journal of Psychiatry* 159, no. 1 (January 2002): 5–11.

31. Emilie Clay et al., "Contribution of Prolonged-Release Melatonin and Anti-Benzodiazepine Campaigns to the Reduction of Benzodiazepine and Z-drugs Consumption in Nine European Countries," *European Journal of Clinical Pharmacology* 69, no. 4 (April 2013): 1–10.

32. Damien Leger, Moshe Laudon, and Nava Zisapel, "Nocturnal 6-Sulfatoxymelatonin Excretion in Insomnia and Its Relation to the Response to Melatonin Replacement Therapy," *American Journal of Medicine* 116, no. 2 (January 15, 2004): 91–95.

33. Michel A. Paul et al., "Sleep-Inducing Pharmaceuticals: A Comparison of Melatonin, Zaleplon, Zopiclone, and Temazepam," *Aviation, Space, and Environmental Medicine* 75 (June 2004): 512–19.

34. Patrick Lemoine et al., "Prolonged-Release Melatonin Improves Sleep Quality and Morning Alertness in Insomnia Patients Aged 55 Years and Older and Has No Withdrawal Effects," *Sleep Research* 16, no. 4 (December 2007): 372–80.

35. Tracy Leigh Signal et al., "Scheduled Napping as a Countermeasure to Sleepiness in Air Traffic Controllers," *Journal of Sleep Research* 18, no. 1 (March 2009): 11–19.

## Chapter 11: Digital Distraction

1. David Strayer, Frank Drews, and Dennis Crouch, "A Comparison of the Cell Phone Driver and the Drunk Driver," *Human Factors* 48, no. 2 (Summer 2006): 381–91.

2. Paul E. Dux et al., "Training Improves Multitasking Performance by Increasing the Speed of Information Processing in Human Prefrontal Cortex," *Neuron* 63, no. 1 (July 16, 2009): 127–38.

3. Joshua S. Rubinstein, David E. Meyer, and Jeffrey E. Evans, "Executive Control of Cognitive Processes in Task Switching," *Journal of Experimental Psychology: Human Perception and Performance* 27, no. 4 (August 2001): 763–97.

4.  Eyal Ophir, Clifford Nass, and Anthony Wagner, "Cognitive Control in Media Multitaskers," *Proceedings of the National Academy of Sciences of the United States of America* 106, no. 37 (September 15, 2009): 15583–87.

5.  Yi-Yuan Tang et al., "Short-Term Meditation Training Improves Attention and Self-Regulation," *Proceedings of the National Academy of Sciences* 104, no. 43 (October 23, 2007): 17152–56.

6.  Anthony B. Newberg et al., "Meditation Effects on Cognitive Function and Cerebral Blood Flow in Subjects with Memory Loss: A Preliminary Study," *Journal of Alzheimers Disease* 20, no. 2 (2010): 517–26.

7.  Tara C. Marshall, "Facebook Surveillance of Former Romantic Partners: Associations with PostBreakup Recovery and Personal Growth," *Cyberpsychology, Behavior, and Social Networking* 15, no. 10 (October 2012): 521–26.

8.  Linda A. Henkel, "Point-and-Shoot Memories, The Influence of Taking Photos on Memory for a Museum Tour," *Psychological Science* (December 5, 2013): http://pss.sagepub.com/content/early/2013/12/04/0956797613504438.abstract.

9.  Ethan Kross et al., "Facebook Use Predicts Declines in Subjective Well-Being in Young Adults," *PLOS One* (August 14, 2013): http://www.plosone.org/article/info%3Adoi%2F10.1371%2Fjournal.pone.0069841.

## Chapter 12: An Epidemic of Loneliness

1.  John T. Cacioppo et al., "Loneliness as a Specific Risk Factor for Depressive Symptoms: Cross-sectional and Longitudinal Analyses," *Psychology and Aging* 21, no. 1 (March 2006): 140–51.

2.  Jonathan Price, Victoria Cole, and Guy M. Goodwin, "Emotional Side Effects of Selective Serotonin Reuptake Inhibitors: Qualitative Study," *The British Journal of Psychiatry* 195 (2009): 211–17.

3.  John T. Cacioppo and Louise C. Hawkley, "Perceived Social Isolation and Cognition," *Trends in Cognitive Sciences* 13, no. 10 (October 2009): 447–54.

4.  Julianne Holt-Lunstad, Timothy B. Smith, and J. Bradley Layton, "Social Relationships and Mortality Risk: A Meta-analytic Review," *PLOS Medicine* (July 27, 2010): http://www.plosmedicine.org/article/info%3Adoi%2F10.1371%2Fjournal.pmed.1000316.

5.  Patricia Sias and Heidi Bartoo, "Friendship, Social Support, and Health," *Low-Cost Approaches to Promote Physical and Mental Health: Theory, Research, and Practice* (New York: Springer Science + Business Media, 2007).

6.  David Myers, "The Funds, Friends, and Faith of Happy People," *American Psychologist* 55, no. 1 (January 2000): 56–67.

7.   S. Ebrahim et al., "Sexual Intercourse and Risk of Ischaemic Stroke and Coronary Heart Disease: The Caerphilly Study," *Journal of Epidemiology and Community Health* 56, no. 2 (February 2002): 99–102.

8.   X. H. Hu et al., "Incidence and Duration of Side Effects and Those Rated as Bothersome with Selective Serotonin Reuptake Inhibitor Treatment for Depression: Patient Report Versus Physician Estimate," *Journal of Clinical Psychiatry* 65, no. 7 (July 2004): 959–65.

9.   Benjamin Cornwell, Edward O. Laumann, and L. Philip Schumm, "The Social Connectedness of Older Adults: A National Profile," *American Sociological Review* 73, no. 2 (2008): 185–203.

10.  Daniel W. Russell, "UCLA Loneliness Scale (Version 3): Reliability, Validity, and Factor Structure," *Journal of Personality Assessment* 66, no. 1 (February 1996): 20–40.

11.  Miller McPherson, Lynn Smith-Lovin, and Matthew E. Brashears, "Social Isolation in America: Changes in Core Discussion Networks Over Two Decades," *American Sociological Review* 71, no. 3 (January 2006): 353–75.

12.  Kross et al., "Facebook Use Predicts Declines in Subjective Well-Being in Young Adults."

13.  Robert S. Wilson et al., "Loneliness and Risk of Alzheimer Disease," *JAMA Psychiatry* 64, no. 2 (February 2007): 234–40.

14.  Alan J. Gow et al., "Social Support and Successful Aging: Investigating the Relationships Between Lifetime Cognitive Change and Life Satisfaction," *Journal of Individual Differences* 28 (2007): 103–15.

## Chapter 13: Spiritual Starvation

1.   Gerrit de Niet et al., "Music-Assisted Relaxation to Improve Sleep Quality: Meta-analysis," *Journal of Advanced Nursing* 65, no. 7 (July 2009): 1356–64.

2.   Myers, "The Funds, Friends, and Faith of Happy People."

3.   R. H. Gillum and D. D. Ingram, "Frequency of Attendance at Religious Services, Hypertension, and Blood Pressure: the Third National Health and Nutrition Examination Survey," *Psychosomatic Medicine* 68, no. 3 (May–June 2006): 382–85.

4.   Kevin J. Flannelly et al., "Belief in Life After Death and Mental Health: Findings from a National Survey," *The Journal of Nervous and Mental Disease* 194, no. 7 (July 2006): 524–29.

5.   Pew Research, "'Nones' on the Rise," Pew Research Religion and Public Life Project (October 9, 2012): http://www.pewforum.org/2012/10/09/nones-on-the-rise/.

# Endnotes

6.  L. Bernardi et al., "Effect of Rosary Prayer and Yoga Mantras on Autonomic Cardiovascular Rhythms: Comparative Study," *British Medical Journal* 323, no. 7327 (December 2001): 1446–49.

7.  Andrew Newberg et al., "Cerebral Blood Flow During Meditative Prayer: Preliminary Findings and Methodological Issues," *Perceptual and Motor Skills* 97, no. 2 (October 2003): 625–30; Andrew Newberg and Mark Waldman, *How God Changes Your Brain* (New York: Ballantine Books, 2009): 48.

8.  Andrew Newberg et al., "Meditation Effects on Cognitive Function and Cerebral Blood Flow in Subjects with Memory Loss: A Preliminary Study," *Journal of Alzheimer's Disease* 20, no. 2 (2010): 517–26.

9.  Linda Witek-Janusek et al., "Effect of Mindfulness Based Stress Reduction on Immune Function, Quality of Life and Coping in Women Newly Diagnosed with Early Stage Breast Cancer," *Brain, Behavior, and Immunity* 22, no. 6 (August 2008): 969–81; Anna M. Tacón et al., "Mindfulness Meditation, Anxiety Reduction, and Heart Disease: A Pilot Study," *Family and Community Health* 26, no. 1 (January-March 2003): 25–33; V. David Creswell et al., "Mindfulness Meditation Training Effects on CD4+T Lymphocytes in HIV-1 Infected Adults: A Small Randomized Controlled Trial," *Brain Behavior and Immunity* 23, no. 2 (February 2009): 184–88; Jason C. Ong, Shauna L. Shapiro, and Rachel Manber, "Combining Mindfulness Meditation with Cognitive-Behavior Therapy for Insomnia: A Treatment-Development Study," *Behavior Therapy* 39, no. 2 (June 2008): 171–82; Sarah Bowen et al., "Mindfulness Meditation and Substance Use in an Incarcerated Population," *Psychology of Addictive Behaviors* 20, no. 3 (September 2006): 343–47; Lidia Zylowska et al., "Mindfulness Meditation Training in Adults and Adolescents with ADHD: A Feasibility Study," *Journal of Attention Disorders* 11, no. 6 (May 2008): 737–46; Istvan Schreiner and James P. Malcolm, "The Benefits of Mindfulness Meditation: Changes in Emotional States of Depression, Anxiety, and Stress," *Behaviour Change* 25, no. 3 (September 2008): 156–68.

10. Thomas Juster, Frank Stafford, and Hiromi Ono, *Changing Times of American Youth: 1981–2003* (Ann Arbor, MI: University of Michigan Institute for Social Research, 2004): 1–15.

11. Rita Berto, "Exposure to Restorative Environments Helps Restore Attentional Capacity," *Journal of Environmental Psychology* 25, no. 3 (September 2005): 249–59.

12. Ruth Ann Atchley, David L. Strayer, and Paul Atchley, "Creativity in the Wild: Improving Creative Reasoning through Immersion in Natural Settings," *PLOS One* (December 12, 2012): http://www.plosone.org/article/info%3Adoi%2F10.1371%2Fjournal.pone.0051474.

## PART V: SPECIAL CARE FOR SPECIAL CASES

## Chapter 14: Mommy Brain

1.  Katharine Sharp, Peter M. Brindle, and Gillian M. Turner, "Memory Loss During Pregnancy," *British Journal of Obstetrics and Gynaecology* 100, no. 3 (March 1993): 209–15.

2.  J. Galen Buckwalter et al., "Pregnancy, the Postpartum, and Steroid Hormones: Effects on Cognition and Mood," *Psychoneuroendocrinology* 24, no. 1 (July 1999): 69–84.

3.  Pilyoung Kim et al., "The Plasticity of Human Maternal Brain: Longitudinal Changes in Brain Anatomy During the Early Postpartum Period," *Behavioral Neuroscience* 124, no. 5 (October 2010): 695–700.

4.  Joseph R. Hibbeln et al., "Maternal Seafood Consumption in Pregnancy and Neurodevelopmental Outcomes in Childhood (ALSPAC Study): An Observational Cohort Study," *Lancet* 369, no. 9561 (February 17, 2007): 578–85.

5.  Joseph R. Hibbeln, "Seafood Consumption, the DHA Content of Mothers' Milk and Prevalence Rates of Postpartum Depression: A Cross-National, Ecological Analysis," *Journal of Affective Disorders* 69, nos. 1–3 (May 2002): 15–29.

6.  Angus Deaton and Arthur A. Stone, "Evaluative and Hedonic Wellbeing Among Those with and without Children at Home," *Proceedings of the National Academy of Sciences of the United States of America* 111, no. 4 (2014): 1328–33.

## Chapter 15: Senior Moments

1.  Archana Singh-Manoux et al., "Timing of Onset of Cognitive Decline: Results from Whitehall II Prospective Cohort Study," *British Medical Journal* 344 (January 5, 2012): http://www.bmj.com/content/344/bmj.d7622.

2.  K. P. Riley et al., "Early Life Linguistic Ability, Late Life Cognitive Function, and Neuropathology: Findings from the Nun Study," *Neurobiology and Aging* 26, no. 3 (March 2005): 341–47.

3.  Charles DeCarli, "Mild Cognitive Impairment: Prevalence, Prognosis, Aetiology, and Treatment," *Lancet Neurology* 2, no. 1 (January 2003): 15–21.

4.  Elias Pavlopoulos et al., "Molecular Mechanism for Age-Related Memory Loss: The Histone-Binding Protein RbAp48," *Science Translational Medicine* 5, no. 200 (August 28, 2013): 200ra115.

5.  Ellen Bialystok, Fergus I. M. Craik, and Morris Freedman, "Bilingualism as a Protection Against the Onset of Symptoms of Dementia," *Neuropsychologia* 45, no. 2 (January 28, 2007):459–64.

6.  Joe Verghese et al., "Leisure Activities and the Risk of Dementia in the Elderly," *New England Journal of Medicine* 348 (June 19, 2003): 2508–16.

7.  C. Fabrigoule et al., "Social and Leisure Activities and Risk of Dementia: A Prospective Longitudinal Study," *Journal of American Geriatric Society* 43, no. 5 (May 1995): 485–90.

8.  J. Y. J. Wang et al., "Leisure Activity and Risk of Cognitive Impairment: The Chongqing Aging Study," *Neurology* 66, no. 6 (March 28, 2006): 911–13.

9.  Ana C. Pereira et al., "An *In Vivo* Correlate of Exercise-Induced Neurogenesis in the Adult Dentate Gyrus," *Proceedings of the National Academy of Sciences* 104, no. 13 (March 27, 2007): 5638–43.

10. Robert D. Abbott et al., "Walking and Dementia in Physically Capable Elderly Men," *JAMA* 292, no. 12 (September 22, 2004): 1447–53.

11. Stanley J. Colcombe et al., "Aerobic Exercise Training Increases Brain Volume in Aging Humans," *Journal of Gerontology* 61A, no. 11 (November 2006): 1166–70.

12. K. I. Erickson et al., "Physical Activity Predicts Gray Matter Volume in Late Adulthood," *Neurology* 75, no. 16 Oct 19, 2010; 75(16): 1415–22.

13. R. A. Whitmer et al., "Central Obesity and Increased Risk of Dementia More than Three Decades Later," *Neurology* 71, no. 14 (September 30, 2008): 1057–64.

14. J. B. Deakin et al., "Paroxetine Does Not Improve Symptoms and Impairs Cognition Function in Frontotemporal Dementia: A Double-Blind Randomized Controlled Trial," *Psychopharmacology* 172 (2004): 400–8.

15. Susanne M. Jaeggi et al., "Improving Fluid Intelligence with Training on Working Memory," *Proceedings of the National Academy of Sciences* 105, no. 19 (May 13, 2008): http://www.pnas.org/content/early/2008/04/25/0801268105.abstract; Susanne M. Jaeggi et al., "The Relationship Between N-back Performance and Matrix Reasoning—Implications for Training and Transfer," *Intelligence* 38, no. 6 (November–December 2010): 625–35.

16. Martin Buschkuehl et al., "Impact of Working Memory Training on Memory Performance in Old-Old Adults," *Psychology of Aging* 23, no. 4 (December 2008): 743–53.

17. Nicolaos Scarmeas et al., "Mediterranean Diet and Mild Cognitive Impairment," *Archives of Neurology* 66, no. 2 (February 2009): 216–25.

18. Elizabeth E. Devore et al., "Dietary Intakes of Berries and Flavonoids in Relation to Cognitive Decline," *Annals of Neurology* 72, no. 1 (July 2012): 135–43.

19. J. A. Joseph et al., "Blueberry Supplementation Enhances Signaling and Prevents Behavioral Deficits in an Alzheimer Disease Model," *Nutritional Neuroscience* 6, no. 3 (June 2003): 153–62.

20. Rachel L. Galli et al., "Blueberry Supplemented Diet Reverses Age-Related Decline in Hippocampal HSP70 Neuroprotection," *Neurobiology of Aging* 27, no. 2 (February 2006): 344–50.

21. A. Veronica Witte et al., "Long-Chain Omega-3 Fatty Acids Improve Brain Function and Structure in Older Adults," *Cerebral Cortex* 24, no. 11 (November 2014): 3059–68.

22. Kathryn P. Riley et al., "Early Life Linguistic Ability, Late Life Cognitive Function, and Neuropathology: Findings from the Nun Study," *Neurobiology and Aging* 26, no. 3 (March 2005): 341–47; Rajesh Narendran et al., "Improved Working Memory but No Effect on Striatal Vesicular Monoamine Transporter Type 2 after Omega-3 Polyunsaturated Fatty Acid Supplementation," *PLOS One* (October 3, 2012): http://www.plosone.org/article/info%3Adoi%2F10.1371%2Fjournal.pone.0046832.

23. N. Sinn et al, "Effects of N-3 Fatty Acids, EPA v. DHA, on Depressive Symptoms, Quality of Life, Memory and Executive Function in Older Adults with Mild Cognitive Impairment: A 6-Month Randomised Controlled Trial," *The British Journal of Nutrition* 107, no. 11 (2012): 1682–93.

24. Laura Zhang et al., "Curcuminoids Enhance Amyloid-beta Uptake by Macrophages of Alzheimer's Disease Patients," *Journal of Alzheimers Disease* 10 (2006): 1–7.

25. Suzhen Dong et al., "Curcumin Enhances Neurogenesis and Cognition in Aged Rats: Implications for Transcriptional Interactions Related to Growth and Synatpic Plasticity," *PLOS One* 7, no. 2 (February 16, 2012): http://www.plosone.org/article/info%3Adoi%2F10.1371%2Fjournal.pone.0031211#pone-0031211-g006.

26. Ying Xu et al., "Curcumin Reverses Impaired Hippocampal Neurogenesis and Increases Serotonin Receptor 1A mRNA and Brain-Derived Neurotrophic Factor Expression in Chronically Stressed Rats," *Brain Research* 1162 (2007): 9–18.

27. Tze-Pin Ng et al., "Curry Consumption and Cognitive Function in the Elderly," *American Journal of Epidemiology* 164, no. 9 (2006): 898–906.

28. Shahin Akhondzadeh, "Saffron in the Treatment of Patients with Mild to Moderate Alzheimer's Disease: A 16-week, Randomized and Placebo-Controlled Trial," *Journal of Clinical Pharmacology and Therapeutics* 35, no. 5 (October 2010): 581–88.

29. M. Moss et al., "Aromas of Rosemary and Lavender Essential Oils Differentially Affect Cognition and Mood in Healthy Adults," *International Journal of Neuroscience* 113, no. 1 (January 2003): 15–38.

30. N. T. J. Tildesley et al., "Salvia Lavandulaefolia (Spanish Sage) Enhances Memory in Healthy Young Volunteers," *Pharmacology Biochemistry and Behavior* 75, no. 3 (June 2003): 669–74.

# INDEX

# Index

# ABOUT THE AUTHOR

**Dr. Mike Dow** is an author, psychotherapist, and the host of shows on E!, TLC, VH1, Investigation Discovery, and Logo. He makes regular appearances on *The Dr. Oz Show, Dr. Drew On Call, The Talk, The Wendy Williams Show, Rachael Ray, Nightline, Good Morning America, The Doctors,* and the *Today* show. He resides in Los Angeles where he is in private practice.

## Hay House Titles of Related Interest

YOU CAN HEAL YOUR LIFE, the movie, starring Louise Hay & Friends
(available as a 1-DVD program and an expanded 2-DVD set)
Watch the trailer at: www.LouiseHayMovie.com

THE SHIFT, the movie, starring Dr. Wayne W. Dyer
(available as a 1-DVD program and an expanded 2-DVD set)
Watch the trailer at: www.DyerMovie.com

□

THE ALL DAY ENERGY DIET: Double Your Energy in 7 Days, by Yuri Elkaim

GODDESSES NEVER AGE: The Secret Prescription for Radiance,
Vitality, and Well-Being, by Christiane Northrup, M.D.

LOVING YOURSELF TO GREAT HEALTH: Thoughts & Food—the Ultimate Diet,
by Louise Hay, Ahlea Khadro, and Heather Dane

MIND OVER MEDICINE: Scientific Proof That You Can Heal Yourself,
by Lissa Rankin, M.D.

All of the above are available at your local bookstore,
or may be ordered by contacting Hay House (see next page).

□

We hope you enjoyed this Hay House book. If you'd like
to receive our online catalog featuring additional
information on Hay House books and products, or
if you'd like to find out more about the
Hay Foundation, please contact:

Hay House, Inc., P.O. Box 5100, Carlsbad, CA 92018-5100
(760) 431-7695 or (800) 654-5126
(760) 431-6948 (fax) or (800) 650-5115 (fax)
www.hayhouse.com® • www.hayfoundation.org

☐

*Published and distributed in Australia by:* Hay House Australia Pty. Ltd.,
18/36 Ralph St., Alexandria NSW 2015 • *Phone:* 612-9669-4299
*Fax:* 612-9669-4144 • www.hayhouse.com.au

*Published and distributed in the United Kingdom by:* Hay House UK, Ltd.,
Astley House, 33 Notting Hill Gate, London W11 3JQ • *Phone:* 44-20-3675-2450
*Fax:* 44-20-3675-2451 • www.hayhouse.co.uk

*Published and distributed in the Republic of South Africa by:* Hay House SA (Pty),
Ltd., P.O. Box 990, Witkoppen 2068 • info@hayhouse.co.za • www.hayhouse.co.za

*Published in India by:* Hay House Publishers India, Muskaan Complex,
Plot No. 3, B-2, Vasant Kunj, New Delhi 110 070 • *Phone:* 91-11-4176-1620
*Fax:* 91-11-4176-1630 • www.hayhouse.co.in

*Distributed in Canada by:* Raincoast Books, 2440 Viking Way,
Richmond, B.C. V6V 1N2 • *Phone:* 1-800-663-5714
*Fax:* 1-800-565-3770 • www.raincoast.com

☐

**Take Your Soul on a Vacation**

Visit www.HealYourLife.com® to regroup, recharge,
and reconnect with your own magnificence.
Featuring blogs, mind-body-spirit news, and
life-changing wisdom from Louise Hay and friends.

Visit www.HealYourLife.com today!

# Free e-newsletters
# from Hay House, the Ultimate
# Resource for Inspiration

Be the first to know about Hay House's dollar deals, free downloads, special offers, affirmation cards, giveaways, contests, and more!

Get exclusive excerpts from our latest releases and videos from *Hay House Present Moments*.

Enjoy uplifting personal stories, how-to articles, and healing advice, along with videos and empowering quotes, within *Heal Your Life*.

Have an inspirational story to tell and a passion for writing?  Sharpen your writing skills with insider tips from *Your Writing Life*.

## Sign Up Now!

*Get inspired, educate yourself, get a complimentary gift, and share the wisdom!*

# http://www.hayhouse.com/newsletters.php

**Visit www.hayhouse.com to sign up today!**

HAY HOUSE

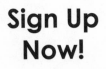
HAYHOUSE RADIO
*radio for your soul*

HealYourLife.com